PUBLIC HEALTH IN THE 21ST CENTURY

PRESCRIPTION DRUG MONITORING

PUBLIC HEALTH IN THE 21ST CENTURY

Additional books in this series can be found on Nova's website under the Series tab.

Additional e-books in this series can be found on Nova's website under the e-books tab.

ALCOHOL AND DRUG ABUSE

Additional books in this series can be found on Nova's website under the Series tab.

Additional e-books in this series can be found on Nova's website under the e-books tab.

CONTENTS

PUBLIC HEALTH IN THE 21ST CENTURY

PRESCRIPTION DRUG MONITORING

CHRISTOPHER J. KAELIN
AND
MEREDITH NUTTING
EDITORS

NOVINKA
New York

For permission to use material from this book please contact us:
Telephone 631-231-7269; Fax 631-231-8175
Web Site: http://www.novapublishers.com

LIBRARY OF CONGRESS CATALOGING-IN-PUBLICATION DATA

ISBN: 978-1-62257-915-0

Published by Nova Science Publishers, Inc. † New York

PREFACE

In the midst of national concern over illicit drug use and abuse, prescription drug abuse has been identified as the United States' fastest growing drug problem. Nearly all prescription drugs involved in overdoses are originally prescribed by a physician (rather than, for example, being stolen from pharmacies). Thus, attention has been directed toward preventing the diversion of prescription drugs after the prescriptions are dispensed. Prescription drug monitoring programs (PDMPs) maintain statewide electronic databases of prescriptions dispensed for controlled substances. This book provides an overview of PDMPs with a focus on supporting access to legitimate medical use of controlled substances; identifying or preventing drug abuse and diversion; facilitating the identification of prescription drug-addicted individuals and enabling intervention and treatment; and outlining and educating the public on drug use and abuse trends to inform public health initiatives.

Chapter 1 – In the midst of national concern over illicit drug use and abuse, prescription drug abuse has been identified as the United States' fastest growing drug problem. Nearly all prescription drugs involved in overdoses are originally prescribed by a physician (rather than, for example, being stolen from pharmacies). Thus, attention has been directed toward preventing the diversion of prescription drugs after the prescriptions are dispensed. Prescription drug monitoring programs (PDMPs) maintain statewide electronic databases of prescriptions dispensed for controlled substances (i.e., prescription drugs of abuse that are subject to stricter government regulation). Information collected by PDMPs may be used to support access to and legitimate medical use of controlled substances; identify or prevent drug abuse and diversion; facilitate the identification of prescription drug-addicted individuals and enable intervention and treatment; outline drug use and abuse trends to inform public health initiatives; or educate individuals about prescription drug use, abuse, and diversion as well as about PDMPs. How PDMPs are organized and operated varies among states. Each state determines which agency houses the PDMP; which controlled substances must be reported; which types of dispensers are required to submit data (e.g., pharmacies); how often data are collected; who may access information in the PDMP database (e.g., prescribers, dispensers, or law enforcement); the circumstances under which the information may (or must) be accessed; and what enforcement mechanisms are in place for noncompliance. PDMP costs may vary widely, with startup costs ranging from $450,000 to over $1.5 million and annual operating costs ranging from $125,000 to nearly $1.0 million. States finance PDMPs using monies from a variety of sources including the state general fund, prescriber and pharmacy licensing fees, state controlled substance registration fees, health insurers' fees, direct-support organizations, state grants, and/or federal grants. The federal government has established two grant programs aimed at supporting state PDMPs: The Harold Rogers PDMP grant, administered by the Department of Justice, and the National All Schedules Prescription Electronic Reporting Act of 2005 (NASPER) grant, administered by the Department of Health and Human Services. The Harold Rogers PDMP received $7.0 million in appropriations for FY2012; NASPER last received appropriations (of $2.0 million) in FY2010. State PDMPs vary widely with respect to whether or how information contained in the database is shared with other states. While some states do not have measures in place allowing interstate sharing of information, others have specific practices for sharing. An effort is ongoing to facilitate information sharing using prescription monitoring information exchange (PMIX) architecture. Currently, there are no national level standards for state PDMP information sharing and interoperability. Legislation has been introduced in the 112th Congress that would take up these issues (see, for example, Section 1141 of the Food and Drug Administration Safety and Innovation Act (S. 3187), the Medicare and Medicaid FAST Act (H.R. 3399, S. 1251), and ID MEDS Act (H.R. 4292, S. 2254)). The available evidence suggests that PDMPs are effective in reducing the time required for drug diversion investigations, changing prescribing behavior, reducing "doctor shopping," and reducing prescription drug abuse; however, research on the effectiveness of PDMPs is limited. Assessments of effectiveness may also take into consideration potential unintended consequences of PDMPs, such as limiting access to medications for legitimate use or pushing drug diversion activities over the border into a neighboring state. Experts suggest that PDMP effectiveness might be improved by increasing the timeliness, completeness, consistency, and accessibility of the data. Current policy issues that might come before Congress include the role of state PDMPs in the federal prescription drug abuse strategy and the role of the federal government in interstate data-sharing and interoperability. While establishment and enhancement of PDMPs enjoy broad support, stakeholders express concerns about health care versus law enforcement uses of PDMP data (particularly with regard to protection of personally identifiable health information) and maintaining access to medication for patients with legitimate medical needs.

Chapter 2 – Statement of John L. Eadie, Director, Prescription Drug Monitoring Program Center of Excellence, Brandeis University

Chapter 3 – Prescribing medications and filling those prescriptions increasingly relies on the electronic collection of individuals' health information and its exchange among health care providers, pharmacies, and other parties. While this can enhance efficiency and accuracy, it also raises privacy and security concerns. Federal law establishes the authority for the Secretary of HHS to develop standards for protecting individuals' health information (which includes Medicare beneficiaries) and to ensure that covered entities (such as health care providers and pharmacies) and their business associates comply with these requirements. The Medicare Improvements for Patients and Providers Act of 2008 required GAO to report on prescription drug use data protections. GAO's specific objective for this review was to determine the extent to which HHS has established a framework to ensure the privacy and security of Medicare beneficiaries' protected health information when data on prescription drug use are used for purposes other than direct clinical care. To do this, GAO reviewed HHS policies and other related documentation and interviewed agency officials.

In: Prescription Drug Monitoring
Editors: C. J. Kaelin and M. Nutting
ISBN: 978-1-62257-915-0

Chapter 1

PRESCRIPTION DRUG MONITORING PROGRAMS*

Kristin M. Finklea, Erin Bagalman and Lisa N. Sacco

SUMMARY

In the midst of national concern over illicit drug use and abuse, prescription drug abuse has been identified as the United States' fastest growing drug problem. Nearly all prescription drugs involved in overdoses are originally prescribed by a physician (rather than, for example, being stolen from pharmacies). Thus, attention has been directed toward preventing the diversion of prescription drugs after the prescriptions are dispensed.

Prescription drug monitoring programs (PDMPs) maintain statewide electronic databases of prescriptions dispensed for controlled substances (i.e., prescription drugs of abuse that are subject to stricter government regulation). Information collected by PDMPs may be used to support access to and legitimate medical use of controlled substances; identify or prevent drug abuse and diversion; facilitate the identification of prescription drug-addicted individuals and enable intervention and treatment; outline drug use and abuse trends to inform public health initiatives; or educate individuals about prescription drug use, abuse, and diversion as well as about PDMPs.

---

* This is an edited, reformatted and augmented version of Congressional Research Service, Publication No. R42593, dated July 10, 2012.

How PDMPs are organized and operated varies among states. Each state determines which agency houses the PDMP; which controlled substances must be reported; which types of dispensers are required to submit data (e.g., pharmacies); how often data are collected; who may access information in the PDMP database (e.g., prescribers, dispensers, or law enforcement); the circumstances under which the information may (or must) be accessed; and what enforcement mechanisms are in place for noncompliance.

PDMP costs may vary widely, with startup costs ranging from \$450,000 to over \$1.5 million and annual operating costs ranging from \$125,000 to nearly \$1.0 million. States finance PDMPs using monies from a variety of sources including the state general fund, prescriber and pharmacy licensing fees, state controlled substance registration fees, health insurers' fees, direct-support organizations, state grants, and/or federal grants. The federal government has established two grant programs aimed at supporting state PDMPs: The Harold Rogers PDMP grant, administered by the Department of Justice, and the National All Schedules Prescription Electronic Reporting Act of 2005 (NASPER) grant, administered by the Department of Health and Human Services. The Harold Rogers PDMP received \$7.0 million in appropriations for FY2012; NASPER last received appropriations (of \$2.0 million) in FY2010.

State PDMPs vary widely with respect to whether or how information contained in the database is shared with other states. While some states do not have measures in place allowing interstate sharing of information, others have specific practices for sharing. An effort is ongoing to facilitate information sharing using prescription monitoring information exchange (PMIX) architecture. Currently, there are no national level standards for state PDMP information sharing and interoperability. Legislation has been introduced in the 112th Congress that would take up these issues (see, for example, Section 1141 of the Food and Drug Administration Safety and Innovation Act (S. 3187), the Medicare and Medicaid FAST Act (H.R. 3399, S. 1251), and ID MEDS Act (H.R. 4292, S. 2254)).

The available evidence suggests that PDMPs are effective in reducing the time required for drug diversion investigations, changing prescribing behavior, reducing "doctor shopping," and reducing prescription drug abuse; however, research on the effectiveness of PDMPs is limited. Assessments of effectiveness may also take into consideration potential unintended consequences of PDMPs, such as limiting access to medications for legitimate use or pushing drug diversion activities over the border into a neighboring state. Experts suggest that PDMP effectiveness might be improved by increasing the timeliness, completeness, consistency, and accessibility of the data.

Current policy issues that might come before Congress include the role of state PDMPs in the federal prescription drug abuse strategy and the role of the federal government in interstate data-sharing and interoperability. While establishment and enhancement of PDMPs enjoy broad support, stakeholders express concerns about health care versus law enforcement uses of PDMP data (particularly with regard to protection of personally identifiable health information) and maintaining access to medication for patients with legitimate medical needs.

INTRODUCTION

In the midst of national concern over illicit drug use and abuse, prescription drug abuse has been identified as the United States' fastest growing drug problem.[1] Seven million individuals aged 12 or older (2.7% of this population) were current nonmedical[2] users of prescription—or psychotherapeutic—drugs in 2010.[3] Over 1 million emergency department visits involved nonmedical use of pharmaceuticals in 2009.[4]

Leading the spike in prescription drug abuse is an "epidemic of prescription painkiller abuse. Nearly three out of four prescription drug overdoses are caused by prescription painkillers" or opiods.[5] Prescription drug overdoses caused 20,044 deaths in the United States in 2008; of these, 74% (14,800) involved opioid pain relievers.[6] Of those individuals who used prescription painkillers non-medically in 2010, nearly three-quarters received the drugs from a friend or relative—either for free, through a purchase, or via stealing the drugs.[7] Aside from prescription painkillers such as oxycodone, other commonly abused medications include benzodiazepines and amphetamine-like drugs.

Florida has been cited as an epicenter of prescription drug abuse. Florida doctors prescribe "10 times more oxycodone pills than every other state in the country combined."[8] Data indicate that 2,488 individuals in Florida died from prescription drugs in 2009[9]—averaging 6.8 prescription drug-related deaths per day. Many have cited the burgeoning number of legal pain management clinics and illegitimate clinics (or "pill mills") as contributing to the epidemic.[10] While Florida has been noted for its legitimate and illegitimate prescription drug distribution, states throughout the nation face the same threats from prescription drug abuse and have taken measures to prevent and treat the abuse as well as to ensure the operation of legitimate prescription drug dispensaries and pharmacies.

Nearly all prescription drugs involved in overdoses are originally prescribed by a physician (rather than, for example, being stolen from pharmacies).[11] Thus, attention has been directed toward preventing the diversion of prescription drugs after the prescriptions are dispensed. Prescription drug monitoring programs (PDMPs) maintain statewide electronic databases of dispensed prescriptions for controlled substances. PDMP information can aid those in law enforcement and/or health care in identifying patterns of prescribing, dispensing, or receiving controlled substances that may indicate abuse.[12]

For over a decade, Congress has provided financial support for state-level PDMPs using electronic databases. In 2002, Congress established the Harold Rogers PDMP grant, administered by the Department of Justice (DOJ), to help law enforcement, regulatory entities, and public health officials analyze data on prescriptions for controlled substances. Three years later, Congress passed the National All Schedules Prescription Electronic Reporting Act of 2005 (NASPER) requiring the Secretary of Health and Human Services (HHS) to award grants to states to establish or improve PDMPs.

The 112th Congress has demonstrated a particular interest in facilitating interoperability among state-level PDMPs, as well as in establishing national programs.[13] While the majority of PDMPrelated proposals in the 112th Congress would focus on enhancing state-level databases and interstate information sharing, others have suggested establishing a national system. A related issue that policymakers may consider is whether PDMPs and their interstate information sharing platforms adequately protect personally identifiable and related health information and whether they can ensure that patients with legitimate medical needs have access to prescriptions. Congress may also exercise oversight with respect to the role of PDMPs in the Administration's action plan to combat the prescription drug epidemic;[14] policymakers may question the extent to which the Office of National Drug Control Policy (ONDCP), along with the other relevant departments and agencies, has taken steps to accomplish these PDMP-related goals laid out in the plan.

This report provides an overview of PDMPs, including their operation, enforcement mechanisms, costs, and financing. It also examines the effectiveness of PDMPs and outlines federal grants supporting PDMPs. Finally, this report discusses relevant considerations for policymakers, such as interstate data sharing, interoperability, and protection of health information.

PRESCRIPTION DRUG MONITORING PROGRAMS (PDMPS)

PDMPs maintain statewide electronic databases of designated information on specified prescription drugs dispensed within the states. Data are made available to individuals or organizations as authorized under state law; these may include prescribers, law enforcement officials, licensing boards, or others. Possible uses of PDMPs include

- supporting patient access to controlled substances for legitimate medical use;
- identifying or preventing drug abuse and diversion;
- facilitating the identification of prescription drug-addicted individuals and appropriate intervention and treatment;
- outlining use and abuse trends to inform public health initiatives; and
- educating individuals about prescription drug use, abuse, and diversion.[15]

In addition to uses of PDMPs aimed at drug abuse and diversion, an explicit goal of PDMPs is supporting access to controlled substances for legitimate medical use. This may best be understood by viewing PDMPs in comparison to earlier, paper-based programs called multiple-copy prescription programs. For example, in 1914 a New York state law required physicians to use state-issued, serialized, duplicate prescription forms for certain drugs.[16] Similarly, California began a multiple-copy prescription program using triplicate forms for specified narcotics in 1939; it expanded to monitor all schedule II narcotics in 1972 and schedule II non-narcotics in 1981.[17] Studies of multiple-copy prescription programs found that many prescribers did not order the required prescription forms, rendering them unable to prescribe specified controlled substances even when medically appropriate.[18] In addition, the ability to check a patient's prescription history using an electronic PDMP might give prescribers more confidence when considering the use of drugs with high risk of abuse.

As of June 2012, 40 states had operational PDMPs, nine additional states and one territory (Guam) had enacted PDMP legislation (but the programs were not yet operational), and one state (Missouri) had pending PDMP legislation. The District of Columbia has neither an operational PDMP nor PDMP legislation.[19]

Program Operation

The entity responsible for administering the PDMP varies by state and may be pharmacy boards, departments of health, professional licensing agencies, law enforcement agencies, substance abuse agencies, or consumer protection agencies. Of the 49 authorized PDMPs, two-thirds are administered by either state pharmacy boards (18) or health departments (15).[20]

Each state determines which entities dispensing prescriptions for controlled substances are required to submit data to the PDMP. These entities can include hospitals and facilities, sole practitioners, or wholesale distributors, among others.[21] Some states also have statutory authority to require out-of-state, mail order, and internet pharmacies to submit data to the PDMP regarding prescription or controlled drugs dispensed to residents of the state. For instance, if a patient in Alabama receives a prescription for a monitored drug from an out-of-state mail order pharmacy, the mail order pharmacy must report the prescription to the Alabama PDMP.[22] State laws also indicate which schedules of controlled substances are monitored under each program (see text box for a brief explanation of schedules), which information about the substances is submitted, the means by which dispensers or dispensaries submit the required information, and the timeframe under which information is submitted.

Schedules of Controlled Substances

The Controlled Substances Act (21 U.S.C. §801 et seq.) establishes schedules for controlled substances (including drugs), ranging from schedule I (most restrictive) to schedule V (least restrictive). Drugs on schedule I have no currently accepted medical use in the United States and are not available by prescription. Drugs with recognized medical uses are on schedules II through V, with each successive schedule representing a lower risk of abuse.[23]

Access to information contained in the PDMP database is determined by state law and varies by state. The majority of states allow pharmacists and practitioners to access information related to their patients, and some also allow other entities—law enforcement, licensing and regulatory boards, state Medicaid Programs, state medical examiners, and research organization—to access the information under certain circumstances.[24] State laws outline the procedures by which information from the PDMP may be accessed.

With respect to how the states identify and investigate cases of potential prescription drug diversion or abuse, PDMPs may be classified as *reactive* or *proactive*. In essence, "[s]tates with [r]eactive PDMPs ... generate solicited reports only in response to a specific inquiry made by a prescriber, dispenser, or other party with appropriate authority" while "[s]tates with [p]roactive PDMPs ... identify and investigate cases, generating unsolicited reports whenever suspicious behavior is detected."[25]

Interstate Information Sharing and Interoperability

State PDMPs vary widely with respect to whether or how information contained in the database is shared with other states. While some states do not have measures in place allowing interstate sharing of information, others have specific practices for sharing. These practices may be based on factors such as agreed-upon reciprocity between states, or whether a request stems from an ongoing investigation.[26] As of February 2012, 28 states allowed for sharing PDMP information on some level—with PDMPs in other states, with authorized PDMP users in other states, or both.[27]

Researchers have provided states with guidance in creating Memoranda of Understanding (MOUs) for interstate data exchange. Questions that states may consider when drafting an MOU include the following:[28]

- How is the information to be reported?
- How will the information be used by the relevant states?
- What are the guidelines on data retention?
- What are the state responsibilities in the event of a data breach?
- Are there measures in place for conflict resolution?
- What are the consequences of potential data misuse?

In addition, the Council of State Governments has highlighted four areas as central to the success of interstate compacts regarding PDMPs and data sharing:

> **Education**—responsibility of providers, data integrity, training requirements (start up versus ongoing)[;]
>
> **Funding**—state funding, costs of data sharing, costs of operation[;]
>
> **Security and Access**—authorized users, authentication, audit trails, Internet access, vendor security, reporting, privacy, confidentiality, use of data[; and]

Technology—data transfer and exchange, uniformity and standards, cost reduction, compatibility, quality/error correction[.][29]

An effort is ongoing to facilitate information sharing using prescription monitoring information exchange (PMIX) architecture.[30] The PMIX program is intended to enable the interstate exchange of PDMP information, providing information on an individual's prescription drug history across states participating in the information exchange. This information can help identify potential prescription drug abuse or diversion, and can help inform stakeholders such as law enforcement, health and human services, health practitioners, and public regulatory agencies. A state can participate in the PMIX program if it has

- legislation allowing it to share information with other states in real time,
- identified at least one other state as a partner in the information exchange, and
- either (1) established an MOU with their identified partner(s) in the information exchange or (2) ratified the Prescription Monitoring Interstate Compact.[31]

The infrastructure of the PMIX program is based on the National Information Exchange Model, which is a data sharing partnership between all levels of government as well as the private sector.[32] To facilitate information security and data privacy, data are encrypted while passing through "hubs," and no data are actually stored on these hubs. PMIX allows for hubs to exist at the state and national levels, and it allows for hub-to-hub information exchange.[33]

With pharmaceutical industry support, the National Association of Boards of Pharmacy (NABP) has developed a technology platform to facilitate interstate sharing of PDMP data, called InterConnect, which NABP has committed to make compliant with PMIX architecture.[34] NABP anticipates that approximately 20 states will be sharing data using NABP InterConnect by the end of 2012, including 14 that had executed MOUs to participate as of March 2012.[35]

Currently, there are no national level standards for state PDMP information sharing and interoperability. Legislation has been introduced in the 112th Congress that would take up these issues.[36] Some bills would, among other things, examine the current interoperability of state level PDMPs,[37] and others would establish national-level standards for the interoperability of state PDMPs receiving federal funding.[38]

Compliance and Enforcement Mechanisms

In ensuring that a given state's PDMP reflects comprehensive data from all relevant pharmacies, physicians, and other dispensaries, one principal concern is how to ensure that these dispensaries are reporting prescription data to the program. The laws or rules governing consequences for failure to report data are determined by each state. For example, one consequence may be disciplinary action by the appropriate licensing board or commission. Another may be that failure to report information could trigger the PDMP program office to report the lapse in compliance to the PDMP governing agency, which may then refer the information to law enforcement.[39]

Program Costs

PDMP expenses involve startup costs, funds needed to operate and maintain the programs, and any monies used to enhance program operation and interoperability. Overall program costs can entail

- hardware such as servers;
- software to run the PDMP database and ensure information security;
- connectivity such that pharmacies and dispensaries can enter data and such that prescribers and/or law enforcement officials can request and access data;
- staff to administer the PDMP and provide technical assistance; and
- overhead fees.

A 2009 evaluation by the Maryland Advisory Council on Prescription Drug Monitoring assessed existing state PDMPs on a range of factors including the costs associated with establishing and maintaining the programs.[40] The overarching finding was that costs vary widely, with program startup costs ranging from $450,000 to over $1.5 million. Further, based on available data from six operational PDMPs, results from the Maryland Advisory Council's evaluation indicate that annual operating costs range from $125,000 to nearly $1.0 million, with an average annual cost of about

$500,000. For example, the state of Florida estimated that it would "cost $480,000 dollars to purchase and initially operate the system for one year" and that "[a]nnual operating costs after that [would be] $450,000 per year."[41]

The Maryland Advisory Council reported that

> [c]ost variations are affected by the frequency of data collection (e.g., daily, weekly, biweekly, monthly), the use of third party vendors for data collection and analysis, the number of prescriptions written and filled in the state, the number of drug schedules (II-V) and drugs of interest collected, and the use of official forms or other required collection and submission mechanisms.[42]

A 2002 Government Accountability Office (GAO) evaluation of PDMP costs in Kentucky, Nevada, and Utah revealed findings similar to those presented by the Maryland Advisory Council. GAO noted a number of PDMP design and operational factors driving variations in state costs for running PDMPs. Specifically, these involved "differences in the PDMP systems implemented, the number of pharmacies reporting drug dispensing data, and the number of practitioners and law enforcement agencies seeking information from the systems."[43]

PDMP Financing

States finance the startup and operation of PDMPs through a variety of channels. PDMP financing often involves monies from the state general fund, prescriber and pharmacy licensing fees, state controlled substance registration fees, health insurers' fees, direct-support organizations, state or federal grants, or a combination thereof.[44] Guidelines for how states may fund PDMPs are outlined in each state's PDMP authorizing legislation. For example, Oregon's PDMP has a fund within the state treasury. This fund receives monies, in part, from a proportion of medical provider fees. These fees are paid to the appropriate medical board, and the board in turn transmits a portion of these fees to the PDMP fund. The Oregon Department of Human Services, which administers the PDMP, may also accept and deposit into the fund money from a variety of additional sources, including grants and donations.[45]

Some states prohibit the use of certain sources of funding, thus limiting the potential range of funding mechanisms. For instance, Florida law specifically prohibits the use of state funds or funds received—directly or indirectly—from prescription drug manufacturers to support the PDMP. As such, the program receives funding from three sources: the Florida PDMP Foundation, Inc., an organization established in Florida law for the purpose of funding the PDMP; federal grants; and private grants and donations.[46]

PDMP EFFECTIVENESS

The available evidence suggests that PDMPs are effective in some ways for both law enforcement and health care purposes; however, research on the effectiveness of PDMPs is limited, especially in the area of law enforcement. Assessments of effectiveness may also take into consideration potential unintended consequences of PDMPs. Experts suggest that PDMPs have the potential to be more effective.

Effectiveness Research

Research on PDMP effectiveness suggests that existence of a PDMP has an impact on both law enforcement and health care. A 2002 GAO study found that "the time and effort required by law enforcement and regulatory investigators to explore leads and the merits of possible drug diversion cases" declined after PDMP implementation.[47] The study found that Kentucky investigations of alleged doctor shoppers took an average of 156 days prior to PDMP implementation and 16 days after PDMP implementation (a 90% decrease). Nevada and Utah reported decreases in investigation time of 83% and 80%, respectively. These decreases in investigation time do not necessarily translate into less prescription drug abuse.

A 2012 review article summarized all peer-reviewed research articles about PDMPs published between 2001 and 2011, which amounted to 11 articles (not all of which addressed effectiveness).[48] The author concluded that PDMPs reduce "doctor shopping," change prescribing behavior, and reduce prescription drug abuse. For example, a 2006 federally funded study (included in the 2012 review article) found that PDMPs—especially ones that issue reports proactively—change prescriber behavior in a way that reduces the per capita supply of prescription pain relievers and stimulants, which in turn reduces the likelihood of abuse.[49] A study published in 2012 (and therefore not included in the review) found that while opioid abuse was increasing over time, the rate of increase was slower in states with PDMPs than in states without PDMPs.[50]

Limitations of the Research

Research regarding PDMP effectiveness is limited, at least in part, by the difficulties inherent in conducting such research. Challenges in conducting high-quality research on PDMP effectiveness include (but are not limited to) (1) defining effectiveness, (2) accounting for differences among PDMPs, and (3) considering potential confounding factors.

In order to study effectiveness, researchers must first define effectiveness in a way that can be systematically measured as a study outcome. PDMPs are statewide programs; thus, researchers look for outcome measures that are available statewide. Some outcomes that have been measured in research on PDMP effectiveness are shipment and sales of controlled substances, benzodiazepine use in a Medicaid population, opioid consumption, substance abuse treatment admissions, drug overdose mortality, and multiple provider episodes (i.e., doctor shopping).[51] On the one hand, opioid consumption includes both nonmedical use of opioids and medically appropriate use of opioids to manage pain. On the other hand, a count of substance abuse treatment admissions fails to capture substance abuse that goes untreated. Each of these measures presents only a portion of the picture of prescription drug diversion and abuse.

Studies that compare states with and without PDMPs and/or before and after implementation of a PDMP vary in the degree to which they account for differences among PDMPs. For example, despite evidence that proactive PDMPs are more effective than reactive PDMPs, most studies do not distinguish between proactive and reactive PDMPs. Another difference that may influence PDMP effectiveness is in which drugs are required to be reported to the PDMP, ranging from only those drugs with the highest potential for abuse to all prescription controlled substances plus other drugs of concern. Research generally focuses on those controlled substances that are included in all of the PDMPs being examined. Differences in PDMPs over time may also influence effectiveness. For example, some states have transitioned from paper-based systems for monitoring prescriptions for controlled substances to the electronic PDMPs used today. Effectiveness studies have generally not accounted for such transitions over time, classifying two different systems as the same PDMP. Accounting for these and other differences between PDMPs may shed light on factors that influence effectiveness.

Researchers must also consider factors that may confound study results, both when comparing outcomes across states (i.e., those with and without

PDMPs) and when comparing outcomes over time (i.e., before and after PDMP implementation). For example, the baseline rate of prescription drug abuse may vary across states; the authors of the federally funded study noted that the likelihood of abuse was actually higher in states with PDMPs than in states without PDMPs, but that proactive PDMPs inhibited the rate of increase in prescription drug abuse.[52] A PDMP may be part of a larger effort to reduce prescription drug diversion and abuse, in which case other initiatives may be responsible for any change in the outcome. A seemingly unrelated event, such as an economic downturn or upturn, may also affect the outcome. These considerations, among many others, impede the ability of researchers—and therefore policymakers—to draw conclusions about the effectiveness of PDMPs.

Potential Unintended Consequences

PDMPs may have unintended consequences beyond reducing prescription drug diversion and abuse.[53] Prescribers may hesitate to prescribe medications monitored by the PDMP—even for appropriate medical use—if they are concerned about potentially coming under scrutiny from law enforcement or licensing authorities. Studies of paper-based prescription monitoring programs that preceded the electronic PDMPs found that many prescribers did not order the required prescription forms, rendering them unable to prescribe specified controlled substances at all. Their concerns may lead prescribers to replace medications that are monitored by the PDMP with medications that are not monitored by the PDMP, even if the unmonitored medications are inferior in terms of effectiveness or side effects. Studies showed that after benzodiazepines were added to New York's paper-based program in 1989, a decrease in benzodiazepine prescriptions was accompanied by an increase in prescriptions for other sedatives. Individuals whose intent is to use controlled substances for nonmedical purposes may also substitute unmonitored prescription drugs or street drugs for those that are monitored by the PDMP.

Like prescribers, patients may fear coming under scrutiny from law enforcement if they use medications monitored by the PDMP, even if they have a legitimate medical need for the medications. Patients may worry about changes in prescribing behavior, which may limit their access to needed medications. Patients may worry about the additional cost of more frequent office visits if prescribers become more cautious about writing prescriptions with refills. Patients may also have concerns about the privacy and security of their prescription information if it is submitted to a PDMP.

Another potential unintended consequence of a state PDMP is that it may push drug diversion activities over the border into a neighboring state with no PDMP. A GAO study, completed in 2002, found evidence of this spillover across state lines.[54] This concern is one of the reasons interstate data sharing and interoperability have become priorities. Similarly, a PDMP may push drug diversion activities into a neighboring state with a PDMP that does not monitor as many medications. In any of these cases, the effectiveness of the PDMP may be offset by unintended consequences.

A PDMP may also have positive unintended consequences. For example, when accessing information from a PDMP, a prescriber or dispenser may identify a patient who is receiving legitimate prescriptions for multiple controlled substances and who is therefore at risk of harmful drug interactions.[55] PDMPs may also enable prescribers to monitor their own DEA number to determine whether someone else is using it to forge prescriptions.[56]

Potential to Increase Effectiveness

A PDMP is essentially a source of information; its effectiveness depends largely on the quality of the information and how the information is used.[57] The quality of PDMP information depends on its timeliness, completeness, accuracy, and consistency. Expert recommendations to enhance data quality include

- collecting data at the point of sale (in real time);
- monitoring all prescribed controlled substances and other drugs of concern;
- integrating electronic prescribing technology;
- sharing data between states;
- standardizing the content across states;
- identifying the person picking up the prescription (which may be someone other than the patient, such as a family member); and
- linking prescription records for an individual (to avoid confusion if, for example, an address changes or a name is spelled differently).

In order for PDMP information to be well used, it must be accessible. A survey of prescribers found that the most common reason given for not using a

PDMP was the time required to access it (73%); two other reasons—difficult navigation of the web portal (29%) and forgetting the password (28%)—may contribute to the amount of time required to access PDMP information. More than a third of survey respondents (39%) felt that accessing PDMP information would not change their practice for that patient, although research suggests PDMP information changes prescribing behavior.

Relatively small numbers of respondents reported that lack of computer availability (9%) or never having applied for access (11%) were barriers to using a PDMP.[58] Expert recommendations to enhance data use include

- providing easy online access;
- issuing automated, unsolicited reports; and
- increasing participation through education and promotional campaigns.

Experts recommend making PDMP information available for research and public health purposes, which would require permitting access by designated non-prescribers (e.g., researchers and medical examiners). An example of a public health use of PDMP information is to identify patients for enrollment in special programs:

Washington state used its PDMP to select Medicaid enrollees for a Patient Review Coordination Program, which decreased emergency department visits, physician visits, and prescriptions (resulting in an average savings of $6,000 per patient per year).[59] PDMP data may also be analyzed to identify geographic areas where interventions (such as increased law enforcement attention or establishment of a substance abuse clinic) are most needed. Carefully controlled access to de-identified data for research and public health purposes may yield other uses.

Federal Grant Programs for State PDMPs

The federal government has established two grant programs aimed at supporting state PDMPs— the Harold Rogers PDMP and the National All Schedules Prescription Electronic Reporting Act of 2005 (P.L. 109-60, NASPER). The sections that follow provide an overview of each program.

Harold Rogers PDMP

The Harold Rogers PDMP is a discretionary, competitive grant program administered by the U.S. Department of Justice (DOJ), Office of Justice Programs (OJP), Bureau of Justice Assistance (BJA). It was created to help law enforcement, regulatory entities, and public health officials analyze data on prescriptions for controlled substances.[60] Law enforcement uses of PDMP data include (but are not limited to) investigations of physicians who prescribe controlled substances for drug dealers or abusers, pharmacists who falsify records in order to sell controlled substances, and people who forge prescriptions.[61]

The program assists states (including U.S. territories) in the planning, implementation, and enhancement of their PDMPs. This involves

- establishing data collection and analysis systems to bolster the drug abuse prevention efforts of law enforcement, regulatory entities, and public health officials;
- enhancing existing PDMPs' use of data in order to identity trends in drug abuse and sources of diversion as well as increase the number of PDMP users;
- participating in national efforts to evaluate the efficiency and effectiveness of PDMPs;
- implementing and enhancing the interstate exchange of information to prevent diversion;
- assessing the efficiency and effectiveness of existing PDMPs and encouraging other states to implement programs; and
- enhancing collaboration between law enforcement, prosecutors, treatment professionals, medical community members, and pharmacies to create a comprehensive PDMP strategy.[62]

Grant Purpose Areas

States may apply for Harold Rogers PDMP grants in one of three categories: planning, implementation, or enhancement.[63]

- **Planning Grants.** States that do not have an operational PDMP may apply for planning grants of up to $50,000, regardless of whether they have regulations or legislation requiring a PDMP.
- **Implementation Grants.** States with legislation or regulations requiring the centralized collection of prescription drug dispensing

data and/or designating the oversight or implementation of such a PDMP to a state agency may apply for implementation grants of up to $400,000.

- **Enhancement Grants.** States seeking to enhance or expand their existing PDMPs may apply for enhancement grants of up to $400,000.

PDMP conformance to prescription monitoring information exchange (PMIX) architecture is an explicit goal of BJA, and grant funding may be used for implementation of PMIX architecture-compliant hub solutions (among other things).[64]

Appropriations

The program began receiving federal funding in FY2002 through the Departments of Commerce, Justice, and State, the Judiciary, and Related Agencies Appropriations Act, 2002 (P.L. 107-77). While the program itself has never been authorized in statute, funding for the program has been provided to DOJ each year through the annual appropriations process. Annual appropriations information is listed in **Table 1.**

Table 1. Harold Rogers Prescription Drug Monitoring Program Funding (In millions of dollars)

Fiscal Year	Appropriation
2002	$2.00
2003	$7.50
2004	$7.00
2005	$10.00
2006	$7.50
2007	$7.50
2008	$7.05
2009	$7.00
2010	$7.00
2011	$5.80
2012	$7.00

Source: FY2002 data from P.L. 107-77; FY2003 data from P.L. 108-7; FY2004 data from P.L. 108-199; FY2005 data from P.L. 108-447; FY2006 data from P.L. 109-108; FY2007 data from P.L. 110-5; FY2008 data from P.L. 110-161; FY2009 data from P.L. 111-8; FY2010 data from P.L. 111-117; FY2011 data are based on CRS analysis of the text of P.L. 112-10; FY2012 data from P.L. 112-55.

National All Schedules Prescription Electronic Reporting Act of 2005 (NASPER)

The NASPER PDMP grant is a formula grant administered by the Department of Health and Human Services (HHS), Substance Abuse and Mental Health Services Administration (SAMHSA), Center for Substance Abuse Treatment (CSAT).

The National All Schedules Prescription Electronic Reporting Act of 2005[65] amended the Public Health Service Act[66] to require the Secretary of HHS to award grants to states[67] to establish or improve PDMPs. Specifically, NASPER is intended to provide grant support to states to establish PDMPs that will allow health care providers to access prescription history information in order to identify patients at risk for addiction.

It also requires that local, state, and federal law enforcement agencies have access to the database. Of note, however, the grants to states under NASPER are only for the PDMP; they do not fund any substance abuse treatment services.

Grant Purpose Areas

The two objectives of NASPER are to (1) foster the establishment of state-administered PDMPs that providers can access for the early identification of patients at risk for addiction in order to initiate appropriate interventions, and (2) establish a set of best practices for new PDMPs and improvement of existing PDMPs.

Appropriations

Funding was authorized for NASPER beginning in FY2006. The program began receiving appropriations in FY2009. The final continuing resolution for FY2011 (P.L. 112-10) specifically prohibited the funding of NASPER.[68] Annual authorizations of appropriations and actual appropriations are listed in **Table 2**.

In order to be eligible for NASPER grant funding, states must meet certain requirements, such as having legal authority to implement PDMPs. All states that submit applications and meet the requirements receive grants non-competitively.

The amount awarded to each state is defined by a two-part formula:

1) Each state receives a base amount of 1% of the total funding (i.e., $20,000 in FY2010).

2) The remaining amount is distributed according to the ratio of the number of pharmacies in the individual state to the number of pharmacies in all states with approved applications.

Thirteen states received grants under NASPER in FY2010, the last year of funding.[69]

Table 2. National All Schedules Prescription Electronic Reporting Act of 2005 (NASPER) Funding through FY2012 (In millions of dollars)

Fiscal Year	Authorization of Appropriation	Appropriation
2006	$15.00	$0.00
2007	$15.00	$0.00
2008	$10.00	$0.00
2009	$10.00	$2.00
2010	$10.00	$2.00
2011	NA	$0.00
2012	NA	$0.00

Source: Authorizations of appropriations through FY2010 from P.L. 109-60. Appropriations through FY2010 from Department of Health and Human Services, Fiscal Year 2011, Substance Abuse and Mental Health Services Administration, Justification of Estimates for Appropriations Committees. Appropriations for FY2011 from P.L. 112-10.

Appropriations for FY2012 from P.L. 112-74.

Note: NA = not authorized.

Program Comparison

Table 3 provides an overview and comparison of the Harold Rogers PDMP and the NASPER PDMP. Basic information is provided on program legislation, administering agencies, program objectives, performance measures, grant types, authorization of appropriations, and actual appropriations.

Table 3. Comparison of the Harold Rogers Prescription Drug Monitoring Program (PDMP) and the National All Schedules Prescription Electronic Reporting Act of 2005 (NASPER)

	Harold Rogers	NASPER
Legislation	Departments of Commerce, Justice, and State, the Judiciary, and Related Agencies Appropriations Act, 2002 (P.L. 107-77)	National All Schedules Prescription Electronic Reporting Act of 2005 (P.L. 109-60)
Administering Agency	U.S. Department of Justice (DOJ), Office of Justice Programs (OJP), Bureau of Justice Assistance (BJA)	U.S. Department of Health and Human Services (HHS), Substance Abuse and Mental Health Services Administration (SAMHSA), Center for Substance Abuse Treatment (CSAT)
Program Objectives	Help states to plan, implement, and enhance their PDMPs.	Two objectives: 1. Foster the establishment of state-administered PDMPs that providers can access for the early identification of patients at risk for addiction in order to initiate appropriate interventions. 2. Establish a set of best practices for new programs and improvement of existing programs.
Grant Funding	Discretionary, competitive grants with three categories: planning, implementation, enhancement.	Formula grant program in which each state with an approved application receives funding according to the following two-part formula: 1. Each state receives a base amount of 1% of the total funding. 2. The remaining amount is distributed according to the ratio of the number of pharmacies in the individual state to the number of pharmacies in all states with approved applications. The HHS Secretary may adjust the amount allocated to a state, after taking into consideration the estimated cost of the state's PDMP.
Authorization of Appropriations	While the program itself has never been authorized in statute, funding for the program has been provided to DOJ each year since FY2002 through the annual appropriations process.	Authorizes to be appropriated \$15.00M per year from FY2006–FY2007 and \$10.00M per year from FY2008–FY2010.

	Harold Rogers	NASPER
Appropriations	Appropriated $2.00M in FY2002, $7.50M in FY2003, $7.00M in FY2004, $10.00M in FY2005, $7.50M in FY2006, $7.50M in FY2007, $7.05M in FY2008, $7.00M in FY2009, $7.00M in FY2010, $5.8M in FY2011, and $7.00M in FY2012.	No funds were appropriated for FY2006–FY2008; appropriated $2.00M per year in FY2009 and FY2010; funding prohibited in final continuing resolution for FY2011. No funds were appropriated for FY2012.

SELECTED POLICY ISSUES

Role of PDMPs in the Federal Prescription Drug Abuse Strategy

In response to the trend in prescription drug abuse, in April 2011 the Obama Administration released an action plan to respond to the "epidemic."[70] This plan, from ONDCP, outlines four primary areas that may reduce the abuse of prescription drugs: educating individuals on the safe use of prescription drugs and risks involved in abusing them; implementing prescription drug monitoring programs (PDMPs) in the states and encouraging information sharing; developing programs for proper drug disposal; and providing law enforcement with tools to enforce proper prescribing practices and disband pill mills.

As part of this plan, the Administration outlined actions to improve the functioning of state PDMPs and increase interstate PDMP operability and communications. Specific actions offered include

- working with states to establish effective PDMPs and encouraging research on PDMP effectiveness and means to improve PDMP effectiveness;
- supporting the NASPER reauthorization;
- ensuring that the Secretaries of the Department of Veterans Affairs (VA)[71] and the Department of Defense (DOD)[72] are authorized to share patient information with state PDMPs;
- encouraging federally funded health care programs to provide controlled substance prescription information to the state PDMPs (in states where they operate health care facilities or pharmacies);
- potentially reimbursing prescribers for checking PDMPs before writing controlled substance prescriptions to patients covered under insurance plans;

- evaluating programs that require certain doctor shoppers or drug abusing individuals to use one doctor and one pharmacy;
- evaluating the potential for state PDMPs to reduce Medicare and Medicaid fraud;
- issuing a final rule from DEA on electronic prescribing of controlled substances;
- increasing the use of "Screening, Brief Intervention, and Referral to Treatment" programs to identify and prevent prescription drug abuse;
- identifying how health information technologies can enhance prescription drug information;
- testing the Centers for Disease Control and Prevention's surveillance system to generate measures of prescription drug abuse;
- assessing the use of the Drug Abuse Warning Network in the domain of prescription drug abuse;
- expanding DOJ's efforts to enhance interstate PDMP interoperability, particularly though the PMIX program; and
- evaluating existing databases with information on prescription drug access, use, misuse, and toxicity.[73]

As noted, supporting PDMPs is just one component in the overall federal efforts against prescription drug abuse. Research on PDMP effectiveness has yielded sometimes inconclusive results, though research findings suggest that PDMPs may contribute to reduced doctor shopping and prescription drug abuse. As such, policymakers may question the extent to which ONDCP, along with the other relevant departments and agencies, has taken steps to accomplish these PDMP-related goals laid out in the Administration's action plan.

Balancing Stakeholder Concerns

While establishment and enhancement of PDMPs (such as interstate data sharing and real-time data access) enjoy broad support,[74] some stakeholders express concerns about (1) health care versus law enforcement uses of PDMP data, particularly with regard to protection of personally identifiable health information, and (2) maintaining access to medication for patients with legitimate medical needs.

Research has demonstrated that PDMPs save law enforcement officials time in investigations, *if law enforcement officials have access to PDMP information*. Concerns about potential law enforcement uses of PDMP data are expressed by stakeholder organizations representing prescribers. The American Medical Association (AMA), a professional association of more than 200,000 physicians, supports the use of PDMPs and recommends that PDMPs be housed in health-related agencies (rather than law enforcement agencies).[75] AMA further recommends that information from PDMPs "be used first for education of the specific physicians involved prior to any civil action against these physicians."[76] The American Society of Addiction Medicine (ASAM), one of several national medical specialty societies under the AMA umbrella, likewise expresses concern about the use of PDMP data for purposes other than health care: "[L]aw enforcement, the judiciary, corrections professionals, employers, and others outside of the health care system should not be granted access to PDMP data except via the means available to them to secure access to other personally identifiable health information."[77] The fact that PDMPs contain personally identifiable health information raises concerns about privacy and data security. Both AMA and ASAM stress the need to subject PDMP information to the same standards applied to other patient records.[78]

Limiting access to medication for patients with legitimate medical need is a potential unintended consequence of PDMP implementation. The prescription drug abuse prevention strategy of the Center for Lawful Access and Abuse Deterrence (CLAAD), which is endorsed by more than 20 organizations, emphasizes that "efforts to prevent abuse must not impede proper medical practice and patient care."[79] The American Academy of Pain Medicine (AAPM), a national medical specialty society under the AMA umbrella, similarly recognizes "the need for policies that support effective control of drug abuse without harming the appropriate treatment of pain."[80] This concern may be related to fears about law enforcement uses of PDMP information, if prescribers are hesitant to prescribe monitored drugs for fear of becoming targets of investigations.

Federal Role in Interstate Information Sharing and Interoperability

In 2012, Administration and congressional attention to PDMPs has largely focused on enhancing interstate information sharing and the interoperability of state systems. The PDMP component of the Administration's action plan to counter prescription drug abuse includes efforts to improve the functioning of state PDMPs and increase interstate PDMP operability and communications. Some bills in the 112th Congress would build on the current system of state PDMPs by establishing standards for information exchange among states.[81] Others would direct certain agencies to examine the current interoperability among state PDMPs.[82]

While the majority of proposals in the 112th Congress would focus on enhancing state-level databases and interstate information sharing, others have suggested establishing a national system. For instance, some proposals would establish a national web portal through which practitioners who prescribe or dispense controlled substances would be required to enter information.[83] Some may argue that monitoring controlled prescription substances is a state level activity, along with regulation of pharmacies and licensing of health care professionals. Others may note that with the increasing reliance on mail order prescriptions and online pharmacies that deliver across state lines, monitoring of controlled prescription substances may be evolving into more of a federal or shared state-federal activity. Policymakers may debate the role of the federal government in incentivizing, directing, or establishing PDMP interoperability and information sharing standards and programs. Such a debate could take place in the context of other federal, state, and local efforts to reduce prescription drug abuse.

End Notes

[1] Office of National Drug Control Policy, *Prescription Drug Abuse*, http://www.whitehouse.gov/ondcp/prescriptiondrug-abuse. Prescription drugs of abuse are often divided into the categories of *pain relievers* (e.g., oxycodone), central nervous system *stimulants* (e.g., amphetamine), and central nervous system *depressants* (e.g., benzodiazepines). Pain relievers that are subject to abuse may be called *narcotics* or *opioids*. Central nervous system depressants may be further divided into *tranquilizers* (also called *anxiolytics*, used to reduce anxiety) and *sedatives* (also called *sedativehypnotics*, used to induce sleep). The term *psychotherapeutics* is sometimes used to capture all of these categories.

[2] *Nonmedical use* of prescription drugs occurs when the drugs are used without a prescription or solely for the feeling they cause. Terms such as *misuse*, *abuse*, *dependence*, and *addiction* are often used interchangeably with nonmedical use, although each term may have its own definition within a specific context.

[3] U.S. Department of Health and Human Services, Substance Abuse and Mental Health Services Administration, *Results from the 2010 National Survey on Drug Use and Health: Summary of National Findings*, September 2011, http://www.oas.samhsa.gov/NSDUH/2k10NSDUH/2k10Results.htm#Ch2. Hereafter: *2010 National Survey on Drug Use and Health*. According to the survey, "current" was defined as using the drug within the past month.

[4] U.S. Department of Health and Human Services, Substance Abuse and Mental Health Services Administration, *Drug Abuse Warning Network, 2009: National Estimates of Drug-Related Emergency Department Visits*, August 2011, http://www.samhsa.gov/data/2k11/DAWN/2k9DAWNED/HTML/DAWN2k9ED.htm#High6. These are the most recent data from the Drug Abuse Warning Network.

[5] Centers for Disease Control and Prevention, *Policy Impact: Prescription Painkiller Overdoses*, December 19, p. 2011, http://www.cdc.gov/homeandrecreationalsafety/rxbrief/. Hereafter: *Policy Impact: Prescription Painkiller Overdoses.*

[6] Centers for Disease Control and Prevention, *Vital Signs: Overdoses of Prescription Opioid Pain Relievers - United States, 1999-2008*, November 4, 2011, http://www.cdc.gov/mmwr/preview/mmwrhtml/mm6043a4.htm. These are the most recent data available.

[7] 2010 National Survey on Drug Use and Health.

[8] Greg Allen, "The 'Oxy Express': Florida's Drug Abuse Epidemic," *NPR*, March 2, 2011, http://www.npr.org/2011/ 03/02/134143813/the-oxy-express-floridas-drug-abuse-epidemic.

[9] Florida Department of Law Enforcement, *Drugs Identified in Deceased Persons by Florida Medical Examiners*, 2009 Report, June 2010, http://www.fdle.state.fl.us/Content/getdoc/742e2162-c1de-4ecd-bce4-857a32c6f42e/2009-DrugReport.aspx.

[10] Legislation has been introduced in the 112th Congress (e.g., the Pill Mill Crackdown Act of 2011 (H.R. 1065, S. 1760)) that would, among other things, provide specific penalties for operating a pill mill.

[11] *Policy Impact: Prescription Painkiller Overdoses.*

[12] Initiatives countering prescription drug abuse range from prevention and treatment to enforcement. These activities include scheduling chemicals used in certain prescription drugs, supporting public awareness campaigns, bolstering law enforcement, and providing assistance to states—in part through PDMPs. This report focuses on PDMPs.

[13] Legislation has been introduced in the 112th Congress that would take up these issues (see, for example, section 1141 of the Food and Drug Administration Safety and Innovation Act (S. 3187), the Medicare and Medicaid FAST Act (H.R. 3399, S. 1251), and ID MEDS Act (H.R. 4292, S. 2254)).

[14] Office of National Drug Control Policy, *Epidemic: Responding to America's Prescription Drug Abuse Crisis*, 2011, http://www.whitehouse.gov/sites/default/files/ondcp/issues-content/prescription-drugs/rx_abuse_plan.pdf.

[15] National Alliance for Model State Drug Laws, *Prescription Drug Monitoring Programs: A Brief Overview*, August 17, 2010, http://www.namsdl.org/documents/PMPsBrief Overview8-17-2010.pdf.

[16] Scott M. Fishman et al., "Regulating Opioid Prescribing Through Prescription Monitoring Programs: Balancing Drug Diversion and Treatment of Pain," *Pain Medicine*, vol. 5, no. 3 (2004), pp. 309-324.

[17] Aaron M. Gilson et al., "Time Series Analysis of California's Prescription Monitoring Program: Impact on Prescribing and Multiple Provider Episodes," *Journal of Pain*, vol. 13, no. 2 (2012), pp. 103-111.

[18] Scott M. Fishman et al., "Regulating Opioid Prescribing Through Prescription Monitoring Programs: Balancing Drug Diversion and Treatment of Pain," *Pain Medicine*, vol. 5, no. 3 (2004), pp. 309-324.

[19] Alliance of States with Prescription Monitoring Programs, *Status of Prescription Drug Monitoring Programs (PDMPs)*, June 13, 2012, http://www.pmpalliance.org/pdf/pmp statustable2012.pdf. For a map, see http://www.pmpalliance.org/pdf/pmpstatus map 2012.pdf.

[20] Alliance of States with Prescription Monitoring Programs, *Prescription Monitoring Frequently Asked Questions (FAQ)*, 2012, http://www.pmpalliance.org/content/prescription-monitoring-frequently-asked-questions-faq.

[21] Alliance of States with Prescription Monitoring Programs, *Prescription Monitoring Program Model Act 2010 Revision*, http://www.pmpalliance.org/pdf/PMPModelAct Final20100628.pdf.

[22] National Alliance for Model State Drug Laws, *States With Statutory Authority to Require Nonresident Pharmacies to Report to Prescription Monitoring Program*, December 28, 2011, http://www.namsdl.org/documents/ ReqmtofMailOrderandNonresidentPharmaciesto ReporttoPMP_001.pdf.

[23] For more information, please see CRS Report R40548, *Legal Issues Relating to the Disposal of Dispensed Controlled Substances*, by Brian T. Yeh.

[24] Alliance of States with Prescription Monitoring Programs, *Prescription Monitoring Frequently Asked Questions (FAQ)*, 2012, http://www.pmpalliance.org/content/prescription-monitoring -frequently-asked-questions-faq.

[25] Ronald Simeone and Lynn Holland, *Executive Summary: An Evaluation of Prescription Drug Monitoring Programs*, Simeone Associates, Inc., http://www.namsdl.org/resources/ PDMP%20Study%20Executive%20Summary.pdf.

[26] National Alliance for Model State Drug Laws, *Interstate Sharing of Prescription Monitoring Database Information*, February 8, 2012, http://www.namsdl.org/documents/ Interstate SharingofPMPInformation02082012.pdf.

[27] For a map depicting the interstate sharing of PDMP data, see http://www.namsdl.org/ documents/ InterstateSharingofPMPData03142012.pdf.

[28] Alliance of States With Prescription Monitoring Programs and Brandeis University's Training and Technical Assistance Center, *Memorandum Of Understanding: Writing Guide for States with Prescription Monitoring Programs*, funded through a grant (No. 2010-DG-BX-K088) from the Bureau of Justice Assistance.

[29] The Council of State Governments, National Center for Interstate Compacts, *Prescription Drug Monitoring Programs: Interstate Compact—National Advisory Panel*, November 5-6, 2009, http://www.csg.org/pubs/capitolideas/enews/enewsissue38/21stCenturyHandout.pdf.

[30] More information on PMIX can be found at http://www.pmpalliance.org/content/prescription-monitoringinformation-exchange-pmix. A pilot project between Kentucky and Ohio's PDMPs formed the springboard for the larger PMIX initiative. Through this pilot, a PMIX hub server was installed in Ohio, and Ohio and Kentucky signed an MOU for data exchange, http://www.ijis.org/_programs/pdmp.html.

[31] Alliance of States With Prescription Monitoring Programs, *Prescription Monitoring Information Exchange (PMIX)*, http://www.pmpalliance.org/content/prescription-monitoring-information-exchange-pmix. Draft language of the compact is available at http://www.pmpalliance.org/pdf/PMPCompactLanguageDraft2010.pdf.

[32] More information can be found at https://www.niem.gov/.

[33] Alliance of States With Prescription Monitoring Programs, *Prescription Monitoring Program Information Exchange (PMIX) Architecture*, Version 1.0, April 2012, http://www.pmp alliance. org/pdf/ PMIX%20National%20Architecture%20Document.pdf.

[34] U.S. Department of Justice, Office of Justice Programs, Bureau of Justice Assistance, BJA Policy on Use of Harold Rogers Prescription Drug Monitoring Program (HRPDMP) Funding to Support Interstate Data Sharing Activities, May 30, 2012, https://www.bja.gov /Programs/PDMPPolicy.pdf. This supersedes interim policy guidance documentation dated March 21, 2012, and April 17, 2012.

[35] National Association of State Boards of Pharmacy (NABP), *Fact Sheet: NABP PMP InterConnect*, 2012, http://www.nabp.net/programs/assets/PMPInterconnectFactSheet.pdf.

[36] For example, section 1141 of the Food and Drug Administration Safety and Innovation Act (S. 3187, as passed both House and Senate) would authorize the Secretary of HHS, consulting with the Attorney General as appropriate, to facilitate the development of recommendations on interoperability standards for interstate exchange of PDMP information by states receiving federal grants to support their PDMPs.

[37] See, for example, the Medicare and Medicaid FAST Act (H.R. 3399, S. 1251).

[38] See, for example, the ID MEDS Act (H.R. 4292, S. 2254).

[39] See, for example, Florida's PDMP rule states that "Failure to report the dispensing of Schedules II-IV controlled substances will result in the Program filing a complaint with the Department [of Health] for investigation and a referral to law enforcement," Rule 64K-1.004,https://www.flrules.org/gateway/RuleNo.asp?title=Prescription%20Drug%20 Monitoring%20Program&ID=64K-1.004.

[40] Maryland Advisory Council on Prescription Drug Monitoring, *Maryland Advisory Council on Prescription Drug Monitoring Legislative Report*, December 31, 2009, p. 76, http://dhmh. maryland.gov/laboratories/drugcont/docs/Final%20Report%20of%20 recommendations%20by%20the%20PDM%20Advisory%20Council%2012-31-09.pdf.

[41] Executive Office of the Governor, Florida Office of Drug Control, *Prescription Drug Monitoring Program Frequently Asked Questions*, http://drugcontrol.flgov.com/pdmp/ faq.html.

[42] Maryland Advisory Council on Prescription Drug Monitoring, *Maryland Advisory Council on Prescription Drug Monitoring Legislative Report*, December 31, 2009, pp. 76-77. An earlier (2002) evaluation of PDMPs by the Government Accountability Office (GAO) found similar reasons for variability in state costs for PDMP operation. These variations were driven by "differences in the PDMP systems implemented, the number of pharmacies reporting drug dispensing data, and the number of practitioners and law enforcement agencies seeking information from the systems."

[43] U.S. General Accounting Office, *Prescription Drugs: State Monitoring Programs Provide Useful Tool to Reduce Diversion*, GAO-02-634, May 2002, p. 3, http://www.gao.gov/assets/ 240/234687.pdf.

[44] Alliance of States With Prescription Monitoring Programs, *Prescription Monitoring Programs: Funding Mechanisms & Business Models*, National Legislation & Implementation Meeting 2010, 2010, p. 3, http://www.pmpalliance.org/pdf/PPTs/LI2010/PMP-FundingBus Models. pdf.

[45] Oregon PDMP statute (ORS 431.960 et seq.), available at http://www.orpdmp.com/orpdmp files/ PDF_Files/ ORS%20431.960%20PDMP.pdf.

[46] Florida Department of Health, *Funding the E-FORSCE System*, http://www.doh.state.fl.us/ mqa/PDMP/funding.html.

[47] U.S. General Accounting Office, *Prescription Drugs: State Monitoring Programs Provide Useful Tool to Reduce Diversion*, GAO-02-634, May 2002, p. 3, http://www.gao.gov/assets/ 240/234687.pdf.

[48] Julie Worley, "Prescription Drug Monitoring Programs, a Response to Doctor Shopping: Purpose, Effectiveness, and Directions for Future Research," *Issues in Mental Health Nursing*, vol. 33, no. 5 (2012), pp. 319-328. Note: The GAO study was not included, because it was not published in the peer-reviewed literature.

[49] Ronald Simeone and Lynn Holland, *An Evaluation of Prescription Drug Monitoring Programs*, Simeone Associates, Inc., No. 2005PMBXK189, September 1, 2006,

http://www.simeoneassociates.com/simeone3.pdf. This study was commissioned by the U.S. Department of Justice (DOJ), Office of Justice Programs (OJP), Bureau of Justice Assistance (BJA).

[50] Liza M. Reifler et al., "Do Prescription Monitoring Programs Impact State Trends in Opioid Abuse/Misuse," *Pain Medicine*, no. 13 (2012), pp. 434-442.

[51] See summaries of several studies conducted between 2001 and 2011 in Julie Worley, "Prescription Drug Monitoring Programs, a Response to Doctor Shopping: Purpose, Effectiveness, and Directions for Future Research," *Issues in Mental Health Nursing*, vol. 33, no. 5 (2012), pp. 319-328; see also Liza M. Reifler et al., "Do Prescription Monitoring Programs Impact State Trends in Opioid Abuse/Misuse," *Pain Medicine*, vol. 13, no. 3 (2012), pp. 434-442; and Aaron M. Gilson et al., "Time Series Analysis of California's Prescription Monitoring Program: Impact on Prescribing and Multiple Provider Episodes," *Journal of Pain*, vol. 13, no. 2 (2012), pp. 103-111.

[52] Ronald Simeone and Lynn Holland, *An Evaluation of Prescription Drug Monitoring Programs*, Simeone Associates, Inc., No. 2005PMBXK189, September 1, 2006, http://www.simeoneassociates.com/simeone3.pdf.

[53] Most of the unintended consequences identified in this section are discussed in Scott M. Fishman et al., "Regulating Opioid Prescribing Through Prescription Monitoring Programs: Balancing Drug Diversion and Treatment of Pain," *Pain Medicine*, vol. 5, no. 3 (2004), pp. 309-324.

[54] U.S. General Accounting Office, *Prescription Drugs: State Monitoring Programs Provide Useful Tool to Reduce Diversion*, GAO-02-634, May 2002, p. 3, http://www.gao.gov/assets/240/234687.pdf.

[55] Jeanmarie Perrone and Lewis S. Nelson, "Medication Reconciliation for Controlled Substances—An "Ideal" Prescription-Drug Monitoring Program," *New England Journal of Medicine*, vol. 366, no. 25 (2012), p. 2341-2343.

[56] Ibid.

[57] Unless otherwise indicated, recommendations in this section are drawn from two sources: (1) Prescription Monitoring Program Center of Excellence at Brandeis University, "A New Generation of Prescription Monitoring Programs: Adopting Best Practices," presentation at Harold Rogers PDMP National Meeting, Washington, DC, June 4- 6, 2012; and (2) Jeanmarie Perrone and Lewis S. Nelson, "Medication Reconciliation for Controlled Substances—An "Ideal" Prescription-Drug Monitoring Program," *New England Journal of Medicine*, vol. 366, no. 25 (2012), p. 2341- 2343.

[58] Jeanmarie Perrone and Lewis S. Nelson, "Medication Reconciliation for Controlled Substances—An "Ideal" Prescription-Drug Monitoring Program," *New England Journal of Medicine*, vol. 366, no. 25 (2012), p. 2341-2343.

[59] Washington state update presented at Harold Rogers PDMP National Meeting, Washington, DC, June 4-6, 2012.

[60] More information on this program can be found at from the U.S. Department of Justice, Bureau of Justice Assistance, *Harold Rogers Prescription Drug Monitoring Program*, http://www.ojp.usdoj.gov/BJA/grant/prescripdrugs.html.

[61] U.S. Department of Justice, Drug Enforcement Administration, Office of Diversion Control, http://www.deadiversion.usdoj.gov.

[62] U.S. Department of Justice, Office of Justice Programs, Bureau of Justice Assistance, *Harold Rogers Prescription Drug Monitoring Program FY 2010 Competitive Grant Announcement*, p. 1, http://www.ojp.usdoj.gov/BJA/grant/ 10PDMPsol.pdf.

[63] Ibid., pp. 2 – 3.

[64] U.S. Department of Justice, Office of Justice Programs, Bureau of Justice Assistance, BJA Policy on Use of Harold Rogers Prescription Drug Monitoring Program (HRPDMP) Funding to Support Interstate Data Sharing Activities, May 30, 2012, https://www.bja.gov /Programs/PDMPPolicy.pdf. This supersedes interim policy guidance documentation dated March 21, 2012, and April 17, 2012.

[65] Unless otherwise noted, all information in this section on NASPER comes from the text of P.L. 109-60.

[66] 42 U.S.C. §280g et seq.

[67] States are defined as each of the 50 states and the District of Columbia

[68] Department of Defense and Full-Year Continuing Appropriations Act, 2011 (P.L. 112-10 §1815(a)(2)).

[69] U.S. Department of Health and Human Services, *TAGGS - Tracking Accountability in Government Grants System*, http://taggs.hhs.gov/AdvancedSearch.cfm.

[70] Office of National Drug Control Policy, *Epidemic: Responding to America's Prescription Drug Abuse Crisis*, 2011, http://www.whitehouse.gov/sites/default/files/ondcp/issues-content/prescription-drugs/rx_abuse_plan.pdf.

[71] The Consolidated Appropriations Act, 2012 (P.L. 112-74) authorized the VA Secretary to share prescription information with state PDMPs.

[72] According to Department of Defense, *Report to Congress: Medication Management for Physically and Psychologically Wounded Armed Forces Members In Fiscal Year 2011-2012*, RefID: 6-B74CA6F, March 14, 2012, "DoD providers can access PDMPs for controlled substance prescription histories before generating prescriptions for controlled substances.... The military specific response to this challenge includes work by the PharmacoVigilence Center to apply the lessons learned and apply it to the military where relevant." The report does not indicate whether DoD dispensers contribute information to state PDMPs; however, if servicemembers fill prescriptions at retail pharmacies in the private sector (in a state with a PDMP), the prescriptions would be reported just like any others.

[73] The White House, *Epidemic: Responding to America's Prescription Drug Abuse Crisis*, 2011, pp. 6-7, http://www.whitehouse.gov/sites/default/files/ondcp/policy-and-research/rx_abuse_ plan.pdf.

[74] For example, the Pharmaceutical Research and Manufacturers of America (PhRMA)—the industry group representing pharmaceutical research and biotechnology companies—supports PDMPs and recommends assessing their effectiveness and exploring enhancements. PhRMA, *Prescription Drug Abuse*, http://www.phrma.org/issues/ prescription-drug-abuse.

[75] American Medical Association (AMA), *The AMA Equation: Illustrated. 2011 Annual Report*, p. 25, http://www.amaassn.org/resources/doc/about-ama/2011-annual-report.pdf; AMA Advocacy Resource Center, *Drug Diversion and Prescription Drug Monitoring Programs*, 2012, http://www.ama-assn.org/resources/doc/washington/prescription-drugmonitoring-issue-brief.pdf.

[76] AMA Advocacy Resource Center, *Drug Diversion and Prescription Drug Monitoring Programs*, 2012, http://www.ama-assn.org/resources/doc/washington/prescription-drug-monitoring-issue-brief.pdf.

[77] American Society of Addiction Medicine (ASAM), *Public Policy Statement on Measures to Counteract Prescription Drug Diversion, Misuse and Addiction*, January 25, 2012, http://www.asam.org/advocacy/find-a-policy-statement/ view-policy-statement/public-

policy-statements/2012/01/26/measures-to-counteract-prescription-drug-diversionmisuse-and-addiction.

[78] AMA Advocacy Resource Center, *Drug Diversion and Prescription Drug Monitoring Programs*, 2012, http://www.ama-assn.org/resources/doc/washington/prescription-drug-monitoring-issue-brief.pdf; and ASAM, *Public Policy Statement on Measures to Counteract Prescription Drug Diversion, Misuse and Addiction*, January 25, 2012, http://www.asam.org/advocacy/find-a-policy-statement/view-policy-statement/public-policy-statements/2012/01/26/ measures-to-counteract-prescription-drug-diversion-misuse-and-addiction.

[79] Center for Lawful Access and Abuse Deterrence (CLAAD), *National Prescription Drug Abuse Prevention Strategy: 2011-2012 Update*, http://www.claad.org/downloads/CLAAD_Strategy2011_v3.pdf. CLAAD is a 501(c)(3) not-forprofit organization that attempts to foster collaboration among health professionals, law enforcement, businesses, government, and other organizations involved in the issue of prescription drug abuse. See CLAAD, *Overview*, http://www.claad.org/about-claad/overview.

[80] American Academy of Pain Medicine (AAPM), *Advocacy: Affecting Health Care on Behalf of our Pain Patients*, http://www.painmed.org/advocacy/main.aspx.

[81] See, for example, the Interstate Drug Monitoring Efficiency and Data Sharing (ID MEDS) Act (H.R. 4292, S. 2254).

[82] For example, section 1141 of the Food and Drug Administration Safety and Innovation Act (S. 3187, as passed both House and Senate) would authorize the Secretary of HHS, consulting with the Attorney General as appropriate, to facilitate the development of recommendations on interoperability standards for interstate exchange of PDMP information by states receiving federal grants to support their PDMPs. See also, for example, the Medicare and Medicaid FAST Act (H.R. 3399, S. 1251).

[83] See, for example, the Fraudulent Prescription Prevention Act of 2011 (H.R. 1266). The database that would be established by this bill might be considered a federal PDMP, although that term is not used in the legislation.

In: Prescription Drug Monitoring
Editors: C. J. Kaelin and M. Nutting ISBN: 978-1-62257-915-0

Chapter 2

STATEMENT OF JOHN L. EADIE, DIRECTOR, PRESCRIPTION DRUG MONITORING PROGRAM CENTER OF EXCELLENCE, BRANDEIS UNIVERSITY. HEARING ON "PRESCRIPTION DRUG ABUSE"*

Good afternoon Chairman Feinstein and distinguished members of the Caucus. My name is John Eadie. I am the Director of the Prescription Drug Monitoring Program Center of Excellence at Brandeis University (Center). Thank you for the opportunity to appear before you on behalf of the Center to discuss our work on enhancing Prescription Drug Monitoring Programs' ability to impede the prescription drug abuse epidemic. We thank you for the honor of testifying on this critical matter.

I. THE CENTER

The Center seeks to help end the prescription drug abuse epidemic in the United States without compromising accepted standards of pain management or the legitimate prescribing of controlled substances.

---

* This is an edited, reformatted and augmented version of testimony given on July 18, 2012 before the Senate Caucus on International Narcotics Control.

In collaboration with the PDMP Training and Technical Center at Brandeis University, the Center of Excellence provides academically sound and practice-relevant information, evaluation, and expertise to PDMPs and other stakeholders.

The Center of Excellence's base funding is provided by a grant from the Bureau of Justice Assistance (BJA) in the Department of Justice, with funds from the Harold Rogers PDMP Grant Program. In addition, BJA, the Food and Drug Administration (FDA) and the Centers for Disease Control and Injury Prevention (CDC) provide a combined grant for the new Prescription Behavior Surveillance System (PBSS) and the Pew Charitable Trusts have provided a grant to produce a White Paper on PDMP Best Practices. To independently and objectively carry out our mission, the Center does not accept funding, directly or indirectly, from drug manufacturers or others with a financial stake in sales of controlled substances.

This is stated at our website at: http://pmpexcellence.org/content/coe-funding-acceptance-policy

Our work is focused on helping PDMPs and other stakeholders to identify and implement the most effective means possible to intervene in the prescription drug abuse epidemic. Our work includes:

- Identifying PDMP Best Practices, including innovative, cutting edge developments that will increase PDMP effectiveness.
- Encouraging innovative uses of PDMP data.
- Assisting in the deployment and evaluation of interstate PDMP data sharing.
- Advancing the methodology for assessing PDMP effectiveness to identify, improve and extend the applications of PDMPs.
- Analyzing PDMP performance measures and identifying improvements in measurement.
- Analyzing and disseminating relevant information through a clearinghouse.
- Providing support to states and federal agencies.

At the Center, we believe we must improve the methods for identifying and interdicting prescription opioid abuse in order to slow down and reverse this epidemic's ever rising toll.

II. Prescription Drug Monitoring Programs – A Brief Overview

Prescription Drug Monitoring Programs collect from pharmacies information regarding prescriber, pharmacy, patient, and drug information regarding each controlled substance prescription dispensed within their states and, in some cases, prescriptions sent by mail order into their states. The data is compiled in each PDMP's database and then made available to prescribers, pharmacies, law enforcement, health professional licensing agencies, and, depending on the state, to Medicaid Programs, medical examiners, drug courts, drug treatment programs and others. De-identified data is generally made available to researchers and evaluators and patients may see their own data in some states.

The rapid growth in states with Prescription Drug Monitoring Programs, with 49 states now having statutorily authorized PDMPs, is a very significant accomplishment. The majority of these programs have been authorized since 2003, when the Harold Rogers Prescription Drug Monitoring Programs Grant program began. Administered by the Department of Justice's Bureau of Justice Assistance, the Harold Rogers' competitive grant program has stimulated growth and enhancements among the PDMPs.

Funding provided by the NASPER program, as administered by the Substance Abuse and Mental Health Administration, is a formula grant program that has been important in assisting states' PDMPs by supporting their operations.

The continued operation of PDMPs and the significant enhancements called for to address the prescription drug abuse epidemic appear to call for continuation and expansion of these funding programs.

III. PDMPs are for both Public Health and Public Safety

At state and national levels, questions have been raised, i.e. should PDMPs follow a public health model rather than a law enforcement model?

As public health professional with forty-two years of experience, I can say this is a specious question; it creates a false dichotomy. The only way for PDMPs to help effectively interdict the opioid epidemic in the United States is to fully engage both the public health and public safety communities in every state and the nation.

For analogy, can you imagine the major public health initiatives to reduce traffic accident injuries and fatalities without fully engaging law enforcement? How would public health agencies enforce speed limits and seat belt laws without law enforcement?

In the same vein, the opioid epidemic, cannot be resolved without the engagement of the entire public health and public safety communities.

For example, the drug overdose death rates for 2008 varied significantly between states (National Vital Statistics System for 2008). What is important to note is three of the largest states, California, New York and Texas, have some of the lowest death rates; lower than many other PDMP states. Common characteristics of these states' PDMPs include:

- The PDMPs provide solicited and unsolicited reports to Law Enforcement personnel: within the CA State Attorney General's Office, the NY State Department of Health's Bureau of Narcotics Enforcement (26 narcotic investigator positions currently) and the TX Department of Public Safety and to Professional Licensing Agencies directly or indirectly.
- They provide PDMP data to the DEA upon request.
- Reports and investigations have focused on criminal activity, e.g. prescribers selling prescriptions, pharmacies selling controlled substances, organized rings of doctor shoppers, pill mills like Sleep Clinics in the late '70s and early '80s (Quaaludes and barbiturates) and Weight Clinics (stimulants – NY) and Stress Clinics in the '80 and '90s (benzodiazepines)
- The three states have used state issued serialized prescription forms – originally for Schedule II drugs. (TX currently issues a single copy serialized prescription form for schedule II prescriptions, NY currently issues a single copy serialized prescription form for all prescription drugs, CA issued serialized forms until 1/1/2005)
- Reports to prescribers or pharmacists are a recent development in these three states.
- All have been in operation for 3 decades or more

Without law enforcement use of PDMP data, these states could not have kept their death rates at these low levels.

Another specious argument has held that doctors and pharmacists will be unwilling to request data from a PDMP is administered by a law enforcement agency. We have examined that question by looking at the proportions of reports issued by six PDMPS (2007) and found there is no difference, i.e. prescribers and pharmacists request 90% to 96% of reports from law enforcement administered PDMPs and board of pharmacy administered PDMPs.

IV. A New Generation of PDMPs: Adopting Best Practices

To deal with the prescription drug abuse epidemic, the nation needs a new generation of PDMPs: *In addition to responding to others' requests, PDMPs need to proactively confront the epidemic.*

Under the grant from BJA, The Center is responsible for identifying and advancing the use of PDMP Best Practices. The Pew Charitable Trusts have provided a grant to develop a White Paper on this subject, which identifies promising practices and the scientific evidence, both current and needed to support these into Best Practices. High priority practices include:

IV. A. Proactive, Unsolicited Reports

Some PDMPs proactively analyze their databases and, when they identify probable doctor shoppers, they send an unsolicited report to the prescribers and pharmacies. Such reports result not only in reducing the subsequent prescriptions obtained by the doctor shoppers listed in the reports but also in significantly increasing prescriber requests for solicited PDMP data. In addition, there has been a general reduction in prescriptions to doctor shoppers, even for those for whom no report is issued. As of a November 2011 survey of 38 states, only 30 PDMPs were authorized to provide unsolicited reports to providers, and only 16 of them were actually doing so. (COE survey of PDMPs, 2011).

A few PDMPs, analyze their data to identify possible criminal activity or professional misconduct and then provide unsolicited reports to the appropriate agencies. In the 2011 survey, only 8 states were providing such reports to law enforcement and only 7 states to professional licensing agencies.

To stem the epidemic, PDMPs must increase the analysis of data and use of unsolicited reports to law enforcement and professional licensing agencies as well as prescribers and pharmacies.

IV. B. Prescribers and Pharmacists: Requested (Solicited) Reports

Upon request, PDMPs provide prescription histories to prescribers and pharmacists so they can make clinically sound decisions prior to issuing or dispensing prescriptions for controlled substances and can avoid being duped by doctor shoppers. This is generally done by PDMPs providing web-portals through which practitioners may request data.

We need to increase prescriber and pharmacists use of PDMPs. Enrollment of prescribers in PDMPs' online data web portals varies by state, between 20% and 50%. The proportion of prescribers who actually request data reports is somewhat less. Thus it is not surprising that Kentucky, New York and Tennessee passed legislation in 2012 basically mandating prescribers to access PDMP data prior to issuing the first controlled substance prescription and periodically thereafter, with some exceptions. These mandates are more significant than some prior states' mandates for accessing PDMP data under special circumstances.

Given the severity of the epidemic and the reality that prescribers are unable to tell when an individual may be a doctor shopper, such mandates may be increasingly considered by states.

IV. C. Law Enforcement Agencies: Requested (Solicited) Reports

Local, state and federal Law Enforcement agencies are essential users of PDMP data. The relatively lower overdose death rates in California, New York and Texas, demonstrate this. While many states permit law enforcement to request and obtain data for an open investigation, other states have added unnecessary hurdles, such as requiring court orders, grand jury subpoenas, and personal review by a state health commissioner. To stem the epidemic, unreasonable hurdles need to be replaced by a more rational process of providing adequate training for law enforcement investigators, a process in which the agency directors retain supervision and accountability.

IV. D. Health Professional Licensing Agencies

Agencies such as State Medical Boards and State Pharmacy Boards need ready access to PDMP data to investigate potential misconduct and inappropriate use of controlled substances, e.g. self-abuse, over prescribing, and offering drugs to solicit sexual favors. Likewise, PDMPs need to analyze their data and forward unsolicited reports to licensing boards when patterns of possible misconduct are found. This process needs to be automated to the extent feasible.

IV. E. Pharmacies: Verifications Prior to Dispensing

Pharmacies should only dispense controlled substances prescriptions after appropriate verification that requirements have been met. For example, controlled substances should not be dispensed unless a pharmacy positively identifies who is picking up the drug and forwards that person's identifying information to the state PDMP. The importance of this was demonstrated when Massachusetts found that 38% of persons dropping off written Schedule II prescriptions or picking up the drugs were someone other than the patient.

Should mandatory prescriber education be established (which the Center strongly supports), the list of trained prescribers should be automatically checked before a prescription is dispensed. The factors identified in the 2009 GAO report should be reviewed prior to dispensing, including verification that the prescriber is currently licensed and registered with DEA, has no licensure or registration restrictions that would affect controlled substances prescribing, and is not deceased. Likewise, patients known to be deceased should not be allowed to have prescriptions dispensed in their names. PDMPs may help facilitate these verifications. Pharmacies will need to be properly compensated for this new work.

IV. F. Expanding PDMP Data Use to Other Users

If the expansion of the prescription drug abuse epidemic is to be slowed and reduced, then other parties need to have access to PDMP data. Some states permit some of the parties below to have access, but this needs to be regularized and expanded:

a) State's Medicaid agency's unit(s) with legal authority to conduct investigations and utilization review of program services regarding Medicaid program recipients or Medicaid program providers.
b) Appropriate Medicare personnel (only one PDMP currently has legislation authorizing such use).
c) Medical examiners, coroners or others authorized under law to investigate causes of deaths for cases under investigation pursuant to their official duties and responsibilities.
d) Substance abuse treatment providers – to track for drugs obtained without knowledge of the treatment programs.
e) Substance abuse treatment state agencies (e.g. analyzed generic information can assist planning for location of treatment programs).
f) Worker's compensation board reviewers.
g) Drug court judges.
h) Department of corrections' health care professional staff, and probation departments, (if they cannot receive information under law enforcement provisions).
i) The Indian Health Services, Veterans Administration, and Department of Defense health care system (not just their prescribers but also the health care clinical supervisors who oversee prescribing and dispensing within those systems).
j) Health care systems' peer review organizations in order to identify and intervene in prescriber and pharmacist over-prescribing and miss-prescribing as early as possible, i.e. before the practices rise to the level that licensure or law enforcement action are required.
k) Other third party payers' health professional care reviewers - this is not currently being done and will require careful design to protect all data, but given the nature and extent of the epidemic, it appears unwise not to develop means by which PDMPs and other third party payers can meaningfully exchange information.

IV. G. Interstate PDMP Data Sharing

The efforts to establish interoperability between all PDMPs needs to be completed. The Prescription Monitoring Information Exchange (PMIX) Architecture which BJA, the IJSI Institute, and the Alliance of States with Prescription Drug Monitoring Programs have developed provides the basis upon which all PDMPs and the various hubs for data sharing are able to share PDMP data.

V. Prescription Behavior Surveillance System

With funding under a grant from BJA, the FDA and CDC, the Center is establishing a Prescription Behavior Surveillance System (PBSS) with de-identified PDMP data from a diverse group of states. With five states expected to participate in 2012 and ten in 2013, the data will be extremely important for tracking the progression of the prescription drug abuse epidemic and its characteristics, for monitoring and evaluating the outcomes from interventions such as new medical education programs, expansion of PDMP unsolicited reports' use and adoption of other PDMP promising and Best Practices.

V. A. Early Warning System

Pioneering work by the Massachusetts Department of Public Health's PDMP and the principal investigator at the Center has identified an important new function for PDMP data. Using spatial analysis methodology to examine probable doctor shopping when the drug OxyContin was introduced and subsequent years, a rapid expansion of doctor shopping can be seen, beginning in the first year, 1996. Review of data for 2005, shows that doctor shopping for all opioids had become widespread across the state and was concentrated most heavily in five geographic areas. A geospatial comparison to hospital data on opioid overdoses and opioid related deaths shows high rates of overdoses and deaths in these same areas. Had this analysis been possible in prior years, the MA PDMP could have issued warnings before the overdoses and deaths became epidemic. Warnings could be sent to all community, state and national stakeholders including health care practitioners, law enforcement, education, substance abuse prevention and treatment organizations, schools, parent teacher organizations, religious organizations and other groups.

The PBSS will be able to use this methodology for the included states and for other states that send de-identified data to the Center. Alternatively, the methodologies can be shared with states wishing to do their own geospatial analyses.

VI. Third Party Health Care Payers and PDMPs

The ONDCP, in its 2011 Action Plan for addressing America's Prescription Drug Abuse Crisis, called upon the Center to host a meeting with third party health care payers and PDMPs to explore appropriate collaborations. The meeting, planned for December 2012, will include participants from public and private health insurers with representatives from units that develop program policies, administer drug utilization review type programs and investigate fraud and abuse.

The private insurance industry's Coalition against Insurance Fraud has identified that annually all public and private health insurance payers pay an excess of $70 billion for enrollees who abuse opioid prescriptions; more than $24 billion is the private insurers' share. (Coalition against Insurance Fraud, 2007). Workers compensation programs which pay claimants' costs for treatment and rehabilitation following work-related accidents have found opioid misuse to be a major problem. The National Council on Compensation Insurance found that a single opioid product became the highest cost pharmaceutical for Workers Compensation Programs (Lipton, 2011).

The Center is following the Office of National Drug Control Policy's call to convene a meeting with PDMPs and third party payers (ONDCP's 2011 Action Plan to address the prescription drug abuse epidemic). The meeting is intended to open dialogue regarding how PDMPs and third party payers may coordinate activities and work together to interdict the epidemic. The meeting will explore, issues such as how the PDMP data, which includes all prescriptions obtained by a person might be utilized to help third party payers assure that enrollees don't bypass lock-ins or other restrictions by paying cash for prescriptions, thus avoiding third party payers from becoming aware of the prescriptions.

Another topic will be considering with public and private third party payers the value of mandating prescribers to access PDMP data prior to issuing the first controlled substance prescription and periodically thereafter, as a condition of payment.

VII. Mandatory Prescriber Education

A majority of prescribers have insufficient training in the use of opioids and other prescription controlled substances to safely prescribe these drugs.

Such education needs to include training in not only the proper use of the drugs but also the misuse of, abuse of, and addiction to these drugs by bona fide patients; the nature and extent of doctor shopping; the extent of theft, counterfeiting and forgery of a prescribers' prescription pads; and how to access and use PDMP data. As noted above, such training should not only be required but technologically monitored by pharmacies prior to dispensing. In addition, PDMPs should periodically review their databases to assure that prescribers were trained at the time their prescriptions were dispensed; non-compliance should be proactively reported by the PDMP to DEA and the state professional licensing agency.

VIII. Issues the Senate Caucus on International Narcotic Control Might Consider

The Federal Government provides funding for the Medicaid, Medicare, Department of Defense, Indian Health Systems and Veterans Administration health care systems. Involved in the prescription drug abuse epidemic are some of the prescriptions issued by prescribers and dispensed by pharmacies who practice within such systems or who are reimbursed by the systems. Persons enrolled in these systems are experiencing opioid and other controlled substances misuse and abuse, overdoses, and deaths.

Given these factors, does it make sense for the federal government not to require, as a condition of payment, that prescribers and pharmacies request PDMP data prior to issuance of the first controlled substance prescription and periodically thereafter (e.g. every six months) when therapy is continued?

Also given these factors, would it make sense for PDMPs receiving federal funds to provide PDMP data to the authorities that administer these health care systems and that investigate fraud within these systems? For example, such data could identify enrollees who may be at serious risk of overdose or death or be involved in criminal doctor shopping rings, i.e. the PDMPs can identify enrollees who are avoiding Drug Utilization Review, Lock-in or other enrollee restriction programs by paying cash for prescriptions or using alternative third party payers to cover some of their prescription costs. Such data might also allow identification of inappropriate activity by health care professionals that extends from within the federal health care systems and then beyond.

In: Prescription Drug Monitoring
Editors: C. J. Kaelin and M. Nutting
ISBN: 978-1-62257-915-0

Chapter 3

PRESCRIPTION DRUG DATA: HHS HAS ISSUED HEALTH PRIVACY AND SECURITY REGULATIONS BUT NEEDS TO IMPROVE GUIDANCE AND OVERSIGHT*

United States Government Accountability Office

WHY GAO DID THIS STUDY

Prescribing medications and filling those prescriptions increasingly relies on the electronic collection of individuals' health information and its exchange among health care providers, pharmacies, and other parties. While this can enhance efficiency and accuracy, it also raises privacy and security concerns. Federal law establishes the authority for the Secretary of HHS to develop standards for protecting individuals' health information (which includes Medicare beneficiaries) and to ensure that covered entities (such as health care providers and pharmacies) and their business associates comply with these requirements. The Medicare Improvements for Patients and Providers Act of 2008 required GAO to report on prescription drug use data protections. GAO's specific objective for this review was to determine the extent to which HHS has established a framework to ensure the privacy and security of Medicare

* This is an edited, reformatted and augmented version of United States Government Accountability Offic, Publication No. GAO-12-605, dated June 2012.

beneficiaries' protected health information when data on prescription drug use are used for purposes other than direct clinical care. To do this, GAO reviewed HHS policies and other related documentation and interviewed agency officials.

WHAT GAO RECOMMENDS

GAO recommends that HHS issue de-identification guidance and establish a plan for a sustained audit capability. HHS generally agreed with both recommendations but disagreed with GAO's assessment of the impacts of the missing guidance and lack of an audit capability. In finalizing its report, GAO qualified these statements as appropriate.

WHAT GAO FOUND

While the Department of Health and Human Services (HHS) has established a framework for protecting the privacy and security of Medicare beneficiaries' prescription drug use information when used for purposes other than direct clinical care through its issuance of regulations, outreach, and enforcement activities, it has not issued all required guidance or fully implemented required oversight capabilities. HHS has issued regulations including the Health Insurance Portability and Accountability Act (HIPAA) Privacy and Security Rules to safeguard protected health information from unauthorized use and disclosure. Through its Office for Civil Rights (OCR), HHS has undertaken a variety of outreach and educational efforts to inform members of the public and covered entities about the uses of protected health information. Specifically, OCR has made available on its website guidance and other materials informing the public about the uses to which their personal information may be put and the protections afforded to that information by federal laws. It has also made available guidance to covered entities and their business associates that is intended to promote compliance with the HIPAA Privacy and Security Rules. However, HHS has not issued required implementation guidance to assist entities in de-identifying personal health information including when it is used for purposes other than directly providing clinical care to an individual. This means ensuring that data cannot be linked to a particular individual, either by removing certain unique identifiers or by applying a statistical method to ensure that the risk is very small that an individual could be identified. According to OCR officials, the completion of the guidance, required by statute to be issued by February 2010, was delayed due to competing priorities for resources and internal reviews. Until the guidance is issued, increased risk exists that covered entities are not properly implementing the standards set forth by federal regulations for de-identifying protected health information.

Additionally, in enforcing compliance with the HIPAA Privacy and Security Rules, OCR has established an investigations process for responding to reported violations of the rules. Specifically, the office annually receives thousands of complaints from individuals and notices of data breaches from covered entities, and initiates investigations as appropriate. If it finds that a violation has occurred, the office can require covered entities to take corrective action and pay fines and penalties. HHS was also required by law to implement periodic compliance audits of covered entities' compliance with HHS privacy and security requirements; however, while it has initiated a pilot program for conducting such audits, it does not have plans for establishing a sustained audit capability. According to OCR officials, the office has completed 20 audits and plans to complete 95 more by the end of December 2012, but it has not established plans for continuing the audit program after the completion of the pilots or for auditing covered entities' business associates. Without a plan for establishing an ongoing audit capability, OCR will have limited assurance that covered entities and business associates are complying with requirements for protecting the privacy and security of individuals' personal health information.

ABBREVIATIONS

CMS	Centers for Medicare & Medicaid Services
HHS	Department of Health and Human Services
HIPAA	Health Insurance Portability and Accountability Act of 1996
HITECH	Health Information Technology for Economic and Clinical Health
MIPPA	Medicare Improvements for Patients and Providers Act of 2008
PHI	protected health information
OCR	Office for Civil Rights
OMB	Office of Management and Budget

Congressional Committees

The increasing reliance on electronic processes to deliver health care services has the potential both to improve the quality of care received by patients, including Medicare beneficiaries, and reduce costs. In particular, the process of prescribing medications and filling prescriptions increasingly relies upon the electronic transmission of patient information among health care providers, pharmacies, and other entities. This can make the prescription process more efficient and accurate; however, the transmission and sharing of individuals' personal information raises concerns about protecting the privacy and security of that information.

The capacity of organizations that exchange health information to store and manage a large amount of electronic health information also increases the risk that a breach in security could expose the personal health information of numerous individuals. In recent years, a number of entities—including health plans, hospitals, universities and medical centers—have reported the loss or theft of large amounts of sensitive personal information, such as health information. Such compromises can leave personal health information vulnerable to inadvertent or deliberate misuse, loss, or improper disclosure. For example, the Department of Health and Human Services (HHS) reported that more than 5.4 million individuals were affected by a breach of their personal health information in 2010. While information technology can provide the means to protect the privacy of electronically stored and exchanged health information, the increased risk of inappropriate access and disclosure heightens the importance of implementing adequate privacy protections and security mechanisms in health information exchange systems.

The Medicare Improvements for Patients and Providers Act of 2008 (MIPPA) requires us to report, by September 1, 2012, on prescription drug use data protections.[1] As agreed with committee staff, our specific objective for this report was to determine the extent to which HHS has established a framework to ensure the privacy and security of Medicare beneficiaries' protected health information when data on prescription drug use are used for purposes other than their direct clinical care.[2]

To determine the extent to which HHS has established a framework to ensure the privacy and security of protected health information, we identified the department's responsibilities by reviewing and analyzing the Health Insurance Portability and Accountability Act of 1996 (HIPAA), and its implementing regulations, the Privacy and Security Rules; the Health Information Technology for Economic and Clinical Health Act (HITECH

Act); and applicable privacy best practices, such as the Fair Information Practices. To obtain information on the efforts of the department's Office for Civil Rights (OCR) in implementing HIPAA's and the HITECH Act's requirements, we reviewed and analyzed documentation related to OCR's public outreach and guidance efforts, enforcement practices, and HHS rulemakings regarding covered entity and business associate responsibilities and compared those documents to statutory requirements. Further, we interviewed officials from the Centers for Medicare and Medicaid Services (CMS), the Office of the National Coordinator for Health Information Technology, and OCR. To determine the uses of prescription drug use data and the risks associated with the uses of prescription drug data for purposes other than direct clinical care, we interviewed representatives from several covered entities and medical associations, and reviewed academic publications.

We conducted this performance audit from August 2011 through June 2012 in accordance with generally accepted government auditing standards. Those standards require that we plan and perform the audit to obtain sufficient, appropriate evidence to provide a reasonable basis for our findings and conclusions based on our audit objectives. We believe that the evidence obtained provides a reasonable basis for our findings and conclusions based on our audit objectives. Our objective, scope, and methodology are discussed in more detail in appendix I.

BACKGROUND

According to HHS, widespread use of health information technology could improve the quality of care received by patients and reduce health care costs. One such technology, electronic prescribing, can be used, for example, to electronically transmit a prescription or prescription-related information between a health care provider and a pharmacy or to provide other technological capabilities, such as alerting a provider to a potential interaction between a drug and the patient's existing medications.

In traditional, or paper-based, prescribing, health care providers that are licensed to issue prescriptions for drugs (e.g., physicians or others licensed by the state) write a prescription, and calling it into or have the patient take that prescription to a dispenser (e.g., pharmacy) to be filled. In contrast, use of an electronic prescribing system consists of a licensed health care provider using a computer or hand-held device to write and transmit a prescription directly to the dispenser. Before doing so, the health care provider can request the beneficiary's eligibility, formulary,[3] benefits, and medication history. Figure 1 illustrates an example of the flow of information during the electronic prescribing process.

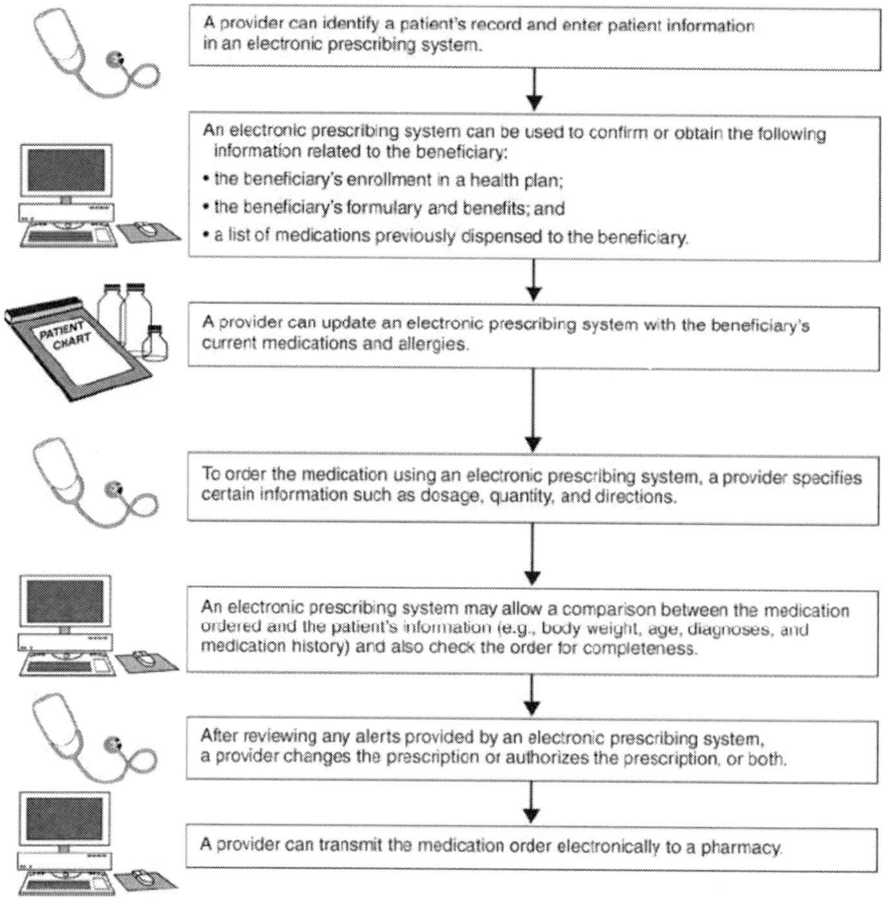

Source: GAO (data); Art Explosion (clip art).

Figure 1. Example of Electronic Prescribing Information Flow.

In order to transmit a prescription electronically, multiple entities need to have access to an individual's identifiable health information[4] in an electronic format. Federal laws and regulations dictate the acceptable use and disclosure activities that can be performed with individually identifiable health information, defined as protected health information (PHI).[5] These activities include treatment, payment, health care operations, and—provided certain conditions are met—public health or research purposes. For example, electronic health information can be held by covered entities[6] that perform treatment functions for directly providing clinical care to a patient through electronic prescribing. These covered entities and business associates, such as medical professionals, pharmacies, health information networks, and pharmacy benefit managers, work together to gather and confirm patients' electronic health information for prescribing, such as a beneficiary's eligibility, formulary, benefits, and medication history. To electronically transmit prescription drug data between a health care provider and a pharmacy, an electronic health record[7] can be used to obtain information about the health of an individual or the care provided by a health practitioner.

In both paper-based and electronic prescribing, information is also provided to the individual's health plan for payment, which would include the identification of the beneficiary, the pharmacy, and the drug cost information. In the case of Medicare beneficiaries' prescription drug data, the information is provided to CMS for Part D payment calculations.[8] Every time a beneficiary fills a prescription under Medicare Part D, a prescription drug plan sponsor must submit a summary record called prescription drug event data to CMS. The prescription drug event data record contains PHI, such as date of birth, the pharmacy that filled the prescription, and the drug dispensed, that enables CMS to make payments to plans. Appendix II provides a summary of the permitted uses and disclosures of PHI.

PRESCRIPTION DRUG USE INFORMATION CAN BE USED FOR PURPOSES OTHER THAN DIRECT CLINICAL CARE

Under certain circumstances, PHI, including prescription drug use information, can be used for purposes not related to directly providing clinical care to an individual. For example, CMS makes Medicare beneficiaries' prescription drug event data available for use in research studies. Release of these elements outside of CMS must be in accordance with its policies and data-sharing procedures. For example, in order to obtain access to this information interested parties must send in an application and submit a user agreement. Table 1 provides other examples of using prescription drug use data for purposes other than directly providing clinical care.

Table 1. Examples of Using Prescription Drug Use Information for Purposes Other than Direct Clinical Care

Use	Example
Research	• The American Medical Association created a quarterly newsletter for primary care physicians, called "Therapeutic Insights," that provides treatment guidelines and prescribing data for specific diseases or conditions. Using de-identified prescription drug use information, each newsletter provides a summary analysis of actual treatment practices for specific diseases or conditions (for example, migraines, chronic obstructive pulmonary disease, and Alzheimer's disease).
Healthcare Operations	• Blue Cross Blue Shield of Massachusetts funded and provided prescription drug use data for a study that estimated the quality improvement and savings associated with medication safety alerts as a result of the use of an electronic prescribing system. The study estimated that medication safety alerts prevented an estimated 402 adverse drug events, and resulted in an estimated annual savings of $402,619 due to lower utilization of health care services. □ A CVS/Caremark representative noted that the company uses de-identified prescription drug use information to predict future use of prescription drugs to benefit inventory management and delivery services. Further, the representative stated that this type of information can also be useful to retailers, who look at these data for inventory management purposes and to anticipate trends for seasonal treatments (for example, flu shots needed for the winter).
Disclosure for Public Health Activities	• Following Hurricane Katrina, a group of public and private organizations launched ICERx.org (In Case of Emergency Prescription Database), an online resource that provided licensed prescribers and pharmacists caring for disaster victims with secure access to a patient's comprehensive medication history. Information accessible on the website included evacuee prescription history information, including drug name, dosage, quantity, day supply, and the name of the provider who wrote the prescription and the pharmacy that filled it.
Marketing	• An official from Verispan, a company that was considered one of the world's leading providers of information, research and analysis to the pharmaceutical and health care industries, testified that the company advertises the use of de-identified data to identify the prescriptions issued by a prescriber and link them with doctor-identifiable data that then can be used by pharmaceutical companies to directly market to a prescriber

Source: GAO analysis of entity-provided and publicly available information.

Depending on the nature of the use, the prescription drug use information is used and transmitted in identifiable form or in de-identified format, which involves the removal of PHI (e.g., name, date of birth, and Social Security number) that can be used to identify an individual.

Federal Laws Establish Privacy and Security Protections of Individually Identifiable Health Information Including Prescription Drug Use Information Used for Purposes Other than Direct Clinical Care

Key privacy and security protections associated with individually identifiable health information, including prescription drug information used for purposes other than directly providing clinical care, are established in two federal laws, HIPAA[9] and the HITECH Act.[10]

Recognizing that benefits and efficiencies could be gained by the use of information technology in health care, as well as the importance of protecting the privacy of health information, Congress passed HIPAA in 1996. Under HIPAA, the Secretary of HHS[11] is authorized to promulgate regulations that establish standards to protect the privacy of certain health information and is also required to establish security standards that require covered entities that maintain or transmit health information to maintain reasonable and appropriate safeguards.

HIPAA's Administrative Simplification Provisions[12] provided for the establishment of national privacy and security standards, as well as the establishment of civil money and criminal penalties for HIPAA violations. HHS promulgated regulations implementing the act's provisions through its issuance of the HIPAA rules–the Privacy Rule, the Security Rule, and the Enforcement Rule. The rules cover PHI and require that covered entities only use or disclose the information in a manner permitted by the Privacy Rule, and take certain measures to ensure the confidentiality and integrity of the information and to protect it against reasonably anticipated unauthorized use or disclosure and threats or hazards to its security.

HIPAA provides authority to the Secretary to enforce these standards.[13] The Enforcement Rule provides rules governing HHS's investigation of compliance by covered entities, both through the investigation of complaints and the conduct of compliance reviews, and also establishes rules governing the process and grounds for establishing the amount of a civil money penalty for a HIPAA violation. The Secretary has delegated administration and enforcement of privacy and security standards to the department's Office for Civil Rights (OCR).

The HITECH Act, enacted as part of the American Recovery and Reinvestment Act of 2009 (Recovery Act), is intended to promote the adoption and meaningful use of health information technology to help improve health care delivery and patient care. The act adopts amendments designed to strengthen the privacy and security protections of health information established by HIPAA and also adopts provisions designed to strengthen and expand HIPAA's enforcement provisions.

Table 2 below provides a brief overview of the HITECH Act's key provisions for strengthening HIPAA privacy and security protection requirements.

Table 2. Key HITECH Act Provisions Related to HIPAA Privacy and Security Protection Requirements

Provision area	Description
Civil Money Penalties	Increases the minimum penalty amount for each violation of the HIPAA requirements. These penalties can extend up to $50,000 per violation and up to a maximum amount of $1.5 million for all repeated violations of the same provision in a calendar year.
Breach Notification	Imposes data breach notification requirements to covered entities and business associates for unauthorized uses and disclosures of unsecured PHI.[a]
Business Associate Liability	Requires business associates to comply with certain HIPAA privacy and security protection requirements.
Use and Disclosure of PHI	Prohibits the sale of PHI for purposes such as marketing without a signed authorization from the individual whose PHI is requested.

Source: GAO analysis of the HITECH Act.

[a]The term "unsecured PHI" includes PHI in any form that is not rendered unusable, unreadable, or indecipherable to unauthorized individuals through encryption or destruction.

Under the HITECH Act, the Secretary of HHS has significant responsibilities for enhancing existing enforcement efforts, providing public education related to HIPAA protections, and providing for periodic audits to ensure HIPAA compliance.

In implementing the act's requirements, OCR's oversight and enforcement efforts are to be documented and reported annually to Congress. These annual reports provide information regarding complaints of alleged HIPAA violations and the measures taken to resolve the complaints. These reports and other related information are required by the HITECH Act to be made publicly available on HHS's website.

HHS Has a Framework for Protecting Medicare Beneficiaries' Prescription Drug Use Information but Has Not Issued Required Guidance or Implemented Required Oversight Capabilities

In response to requirements set forth in HIPAA and the HITECH Act, HHS, through OCR, has established a framework for protecting the privacy and security of individually identifiable health information, including Medicare beneficiaries' prescription drug use information used for purposes other than directly providing clinical care. This framework includes (1) establishing regulatory requirements, (2) issuing guidance and performing outreach efforts, and (3) conducting enforcement activities to ensure compliance with the rules. However, OCR has not issued required guidance to assist entities in de-identifying individually identifiable health information due to—according to officials—competing priorities for resources and internal and external reviews. Furthermore, although it has recently initiated a pilot audit program, the office has not implemented periodic compliance audits as required by the HITECH Act. Until these requirements are fulfilled, OCR will have limited assurance that covered entities and business associates are complying with HIPAA regulations.

HHS Issued Regulations to Implement Key HIPAA and HITECH Act Requirements for Protecting PHI

The Secretary of HHS issued regulations, such as the HIPAA rules, that implement HIPAA requirements and amendments required by the HITECH Act to govern the privacy and security of individually identifiable health information, known as PHI. These rules establish the required protections and acceptable uses and disclosures of individually identifiable health information, including Medicare beneficiaries' prescription drug use information.

HHS Issued the HIPAA Privacy and Security Rules to Meet HIPAA Requirements

HIPAA provided for the Secretary of HHS to, among other things, (1) issue privacy regulations governing the use and disclosure of PHI and (2) adopt security regulations requiring covered entities to maintain reasonable and appropriate technical, administrative, and physical safeguards to protect the information.

Table 3. Key Privacy Principles in the HIPAA Privacy Rule

Principle	Limits the circumstances in which an individual's protected health information may be used or disclosed by covered entities and provides for accounting of certain disclosures; requires covered entities to make reasonable efforts to disclose or use only the minimum necessary information to accomplish the intended purpose for the uses, disclosures, or requests, with certain exceptions such as for treatment or as required by law.
Uses and disclosures	Requires most covered entities to provide a notice of their privacy practices including how protected health information may be used and disclosed.
Access	Establishes individuals' right to review and obtain a copy of their protected health information held in a designated record set.
Security	Requires covered entities to safeguard protected health information from inappropriate use or disclosure.
Amendments	Gives individuals the right to request from covered entities changes to inaccurate or incomplete protected health information held in a designated record set.
Administrative requirements	Requires covered entities to implement a set of administrative requirements, including policies and procedures and workforce training, to ensure compliance with provisions of the Privacy Rule, taking into account their own needs and environment.
Authorization	Requires covered entities to obtain the individual's written authorization for uses and disclosures of protected health information except for certain specified purposes, such as for treatment, payment, and health care operations, or as required by law. Covered entities may choose to obtain an individual's consent to use or disclose protected health information to carry out treatment, payment, or health care operations but are not required to do so.

Source: GAO analysis of the HIPAA Privacy Rule.

In December 2000, to address the privacy regulation requirement, HHS issued the Privacy Rule.[14] The Privacy Rule regulates covered entities' use and disclosure of PHI. Under the Privacy Rule, a covered entity may not use or disclose an individual's PHI without the individual's written authorization, except in certain circumstances expressly permitted by the Privacy Rule. The Privacy Rule reflects basic privacy principles for ensuring the protection of personal health information, as summarized in table 3.

The Privacy Rule generally requires that a covered entity make reasonable efforts to use, disclose, or request only the minimum necessary PHI to accomplish the intended purpose.[15] Further, the Privacy Rule establishes methods for de-identifying PHI.

Under the rule, once identifiers are removed from a data set, it is no longer considered individually identifiable health information and the HIPAA protections no longer apply. De-identification provides a mechanism for reducing the amount of PHI used and disclosed. The Privacy Rule establishes two ways in which PHI can be de-identified. The Safe Harbor Method requires the removal of 18 unique types of identifiers from a data set coupled with no actual knowledge that the remaining data could be used to reidentify an individual, either alone or in combination with other information.[16]

The expert determination method requires a qualified statistician or other appropriate expert, using generally accepted statistical and scientific principles, to determine that the risk is very small that an individual could be identified from the information when used alone or in combination with other reasonably available information.

In February 2003, to implement HIPAA security requirements for protecting PHI, HHS issued the HIPAA Security Rule.[17] To ensure that reasonable safeguards are in place to protect electronic PHI, including Medicare beneficiaries' health information, from unauthorized access or disclosure, the Security Rule specifies a series of administrative, technical, and physical safeguards for covered entities to implement to ensure the confidentiality, integrity, and availability of electronic PHI. Table 4 summarizes these security safeguards.

The Security Rule, which applies only to PHI in electronic form, states that covered entities have the flexibility to use any security measures that allow them to reasonably and appropriately implement specified standards. Specifically, the rule states that in deciding what security measures are appropriate, the covered entity must take into account elements such as its size, complexity, technical infrastructure, cost of security measures, and the probability and criticality of potential risks to its PHI.

Table 4. Security Rule Safeguards

Safeguard	Description	Examples
Administrative	Actions, policies, and procedures that manage the selection, development, implementation, and maintenance of security measures to protect electronic PHI and to manage the conduct of the covered entity's workforce in relation to the protection of that information.	Security management process Security incident management Security awareness and training Contingency plans
Physical	Measures, policies, and procedures to protect a covered entity's electronic information systems and related buildings and equipment, from natural and environmental hazards, and unauthorized intrusion.	Facility access controls Workstation security Device and media controls
Technical	Technical measures and the policy and procedures for their use that protect the integrity and control access to PHI.	Access controls Audit controls Person or entity authentication

Source: GAO analysis of the HIPAA Security Rule.

HHS Issued and Amended HIPAA Rules in Response to the HITECH Act

The HITECH Act set additional requirements for the Secretary of HHS and expanded and strengthened certain privacy and security requirements mandated under HIPAA and the HIPAA rules. Specifically, to implement provisions of the HITECH Act, the Secretary was required to (1) issue breach notification regulations to require covered entities and business associates under HIPAA to provide notification to affected individuals and the Secretary concerning the unauthorized use and disclosure of unsecured PHI; (2) establish enforcement provisions for imposing an increased tiered structure for civil money penalties for violations of the Privacy and Security Rules; and (3) extend certain Privacy and Security Rule requirements to business associates of covered entities. Such required activities are intended to strengthen protections for PHI, including Medicare beneficiaries' prescription drug use information.

To implement these provisions of the act, OCR issued two interim final rules[18]—the Breach Notification for Unsecured Protected Health Information Rule,[19] known as the "Breach Notification Rule," and the HITECH Act Enforcement Rule[20]—and has developed a draft rule intended to, among other things, extend the applicability of certain requirements of the Privacy and

Security Rules to business associates. OCR issued the Breach Notification for Unsecured Protected Health Information Rule in August 2009. This rule contains detailed requirements for HIPAA-covered entities and business associates to notify affected individuals and the Secretary following the discovery of a breach of unsecured PHI.[21] In addition, in October 2009, OCR issued the HITECH Enforcement Rule, which amends the HIPAA rules to incorporate HITECH Act provisions establishing categories of violations based on increasing levels of culpability and correspondingly increased tier ranges of civil money penalty amounts.

In addition, in July 2010, OCR issued a notice of proposed rulemaking[22] to modify the HIPAA Privacy, Security, and Enforcement Rules to implement other provisions of the HITECH Act. According to the OCR website, the proposed rule is intended to, among other things, make modifications to extend the applicability of certain Privacy and Security Rule requirements to the business associates of covered entities, strengthen limitations on the use or disclosure of PHI for marketing and fundraising and prohibit the sale of PHI, and expand individuals' rights to access their information and obtain restrictions on certain disclosures of protected health information to health plans. According to OCR officials, the proposed rule is currently under review by the Office of Management and Budget (OMB), and OCR officials have not determined an estimated time frame for its issuance.

OCR Provides Guidance and Outreach on the Use of PHI, but Has Not Issued Required De-identification Guidance

The HITECH Act also requires HHS to educate members of the public about how their PHI, which may include Medicare beneficiaries' prescription drug use information, may be used. In addition, the HITECH Act requires HHS to provide guidance for covered entities on implementing HIPAA requirements for de-identifying data—that is, taking steps to ensure the data cannot be linked to a specific individual. Specifically, the act requires HHS to provide information to educate individuals about the potential uses of PHI, the effects of such uses, and the rights of individuals with respect to such uses. In addition—to clarify the de-identification methods established in the HIPAA Privacy Rule—the HITECH Act required OCR to produce guidance by February 2010 on how best to implement the HIPAA Privacy Rule requirements for the de-identification of protected health information.

OCR has undertaken an array of efforts since the rules were issued, as well as to implement the HITECH Act's requirements to promote awareness of the general uses of PHI and the privacy and security protections afforded to the identifiable information. For example, the office has made various types of information resources publicly available.[23] Through its website, the office provides a central hub of resources related to HIPAA regulations, ranging from guidance to consumers on their rights and protections under the HIPAA rules to compliance guidance to covered entities.[24] More specifically, the office has developed resources to guide covered entities and business associates in implementing the provisions of the Privacy and Security Rules, which include, among other things, examples of business associate contract provisions for sharing PHI, answers to commonly asked questions, summaries of the HIPAA rules, and information on regional privacy officers designated to offer guidance and education assistance to entities and individuals on rights and responsibilities related to the Privacy and Security Rules. Table 5 below provides a brief overview of OCR's guidance and education outreach activities in regard to their target audience, purpose, and guidance materials. In another effort to promote awareness, OCR—in conjunction with the Office of the National Coordinator for Health Information Technology[25]— established a Privacy and Security Toolkit to provide guidance on privacy and security practices for covered entities that electronically exchange health information in a network environment. The toolkit was developed to implement the Nationwide Privacy and Security Framework for Electronic Exchange of Individually Identifiable Health Information, also known as the Privacy and Security Framework,[26] and includes tools to facilitate the implementation of these practices to protect PHI. Guidance included with the toolkit includes, among other things, security guidelines to assist small health care practices as they become more reliant on health information technology and facts and template examples for developing notices for informing consumers about a company's privacy and security policies in a web-based environment. Although OCR has initiated these efforts to fulfill its responsibilities to promote awareness of allowable uses and provide guidance for complying with required protections under the HITECH Act, it has yet to publish HITECH Act guidance on implementing HIPAA de-identification methods, which was to be issued by February 2010.[27] OCR officials stated that they have developed a draft of the de-identification guidance, but have not set an estimated issuance date. According to the officials, the draft guidance was developed based on the office's solicitation of best practices and guidelines from multiple venues and forums, including a workshop panel discussion with industry experts in March 2010 that included discussions on best practices and risks associated with de-identifying PHI. The officials stated that guidance will explain and answer questions about de-identification methods as well as clarify guidelines for conducting the expert determination method of de-identification to reduce entities' reliance on the Safe Harbor method.

Table 5. Overview of OCR's Guidance and Education Outreach Activities

Target audience	Purpose	Guidance materials
General public	To enable the public to be better informed about the uses of PHI and the privacy protections and rights afforded to the public by the HIPAA rules	• Information on individual health information privacy rights • Summaries of the statutory and regulatory protections of PHI • Sharing information with family members and friends • Notices of Privacy Practices • Videos about HIPAA and individual rights available on the OCR YouTube channel
Covered entities/business associates	To promote compliance with the Privacy and Security Rules	• Summaries of the Privacy and Security Rules • Implementation guidance for significant aspects of the HIPAA rules • Presentations related to HIPAA rules • Answers to frequently asked questions • Examples of business associate contract provisions for sharing PHI • Privacy electronic mailing list to inform entities about the release of newly available resources related to health information privacy frequently asked questions, guidance, and technical assistance materials, as well as other announcements

Source: GAO analysis of OCR data.

The issuance of such implementation guidance could provide covered entities—including those that rely on de-identified prescription drug use information for purposes other than directly providing clinical care—with guidelines and leading practices for properly de-identifying PHI in accordance with Privacy Rule requirements. According to OCR officials, competing priorities for resources and internal reviews have delayed the issuance of the guidance. Officials stated that the draft is currently under government wide review. Although officials stated that the guidance will be issued upon completion of the review, no estimated time frame has been set. Until this guidance is issued, increased risk exists that covered entities are not properly implementing the standards set by the HIPAA Privacy Rule and that identifiers are not properly removed from PHI.

OCR Conducts Enforcement and Oversight Activities but Has Yet to Implement a Sustained Audit Capability

Federal laws authorize HHS to take steps to ensure that covered entities comply with HIPAA privacy and security requirements targeted toward protecting patient data, including Medicare beneficiaries' prescription drug use information. Specifically, HHS has authority to enforce compliance with the Privacy and Security Rules in response to, among other things, (1) complaints reporting potential privacy and security violations and (2) data breach notifications submitted by covered entities.[28] Furthermore, the HITECH Act increased HHS's oversight responsibilities by requiring the department to perform periodic audits to ensure covered entities and business associates are complying with the Privacy and Security Rules and breach notification standards.[29]

OCR Has Investigated Reported Violations of the Privacy and Security Rules

OCR has developed and implemented an enforcement process that is focused on conducting investigations in response to actions that potentially violate the Privacy and Security Rules. According to OCR officials, the office opens investigations in response to submitted complaints and data breach notifications, as well as conducts compliance reviews based on other reports of potential violations of which the department becomes aware. If necessary, it then requires covered entities to make changes to their privacy and security practices.

OCR receives thousands of complaints[30] and breach notifications[31] each year. Officials stated that these complaints and notifications are reviewed to determine if they are eligible for enforcement and require an OCR investigation. According to information provided by OCR, from 2006 to

2010[32] the office has received on average about 8,000 Privacy and Security Rule complaints each year.[33] OCR officials reported that as of February 2012, the office conducted investigations of approximately 24,000 complaints alleging compliance violations of the Privacy or Security Rule, resulting in corrective actions by covered entities in 66 percent of the cases. Corrective actions have included training or sanctioning employees, revising policies and procedures, and mitigating any alleged harm. According to OCR's annual report to Congress on HIPAA Privacy and Security Rule compliance,[34] in instances where an investigation resulted in a determination that a violation of the Privacy or Security Rule occurred, the office first attempted to resolve the case informally by obtaining voluntary compliance through corrective action. Compliance issues investigated most often include impermissible uses and disclosures of PHI and lack of safeguards for or patient access to PHI.

As of May 2012, OCR investigations have resulted in the issuance of a resolution agreement in eight cases. According to OCR officials, a resolution agreement is a formal agreement between OCR and the investigated entity and is used to settle investigations with more serious outcomes. A resolution agreement is a contract signed by HHS and a covered entity in which the covered entity agrees to perform corrective actions (e.g., staff training), submit progress reports to HHS (generally for a period of 3 years), and—in some cases—pay a monetary fine. The eight resolution agreements entered into with the investigated entities all included a payment of a resolution amount, and the development or revision of policies and procedures. In six of these cases further submission of compliance reports or compliance monitoring was required for 2 to 3 years. For example, in response to complaints that several patients' electronic PHI was viewed without permission by university health system employees, OCR initiated an investigation which revealed that unauthorized employees repeatedly looked at the electronic PHI for numerous patients. The university health system agreed to settle potential violations of the Privacy and Security Rules by committing to a corrective action plan and paying approximately $865,000.

When a covered entity does not cooperate with an OCR investigation or take action to resolve a violation, the office also has the authority to impose a civil money penalty. OCR can levy civil money penalties for failure to comply with the requirements of the Privacy Rule, Security Rule, and Breach Notification Rule. For each violation, the maximum penalty amount in four separate categories[35] is $50,000. For multiple violations of an identical provision in a calendar year, the maximum penalty in each category is $1.5 million. As of May 2012, OCR had issued one civil money penalty for noncompliance in the amount of $4.3 million. Since February 2010, pursuant to the HITECH Act, OCR has received and used the money from settlement amounts and civil money penalties for enforcement of the HIPAA rules.

OCR Has Not Developed a Sustained Audit Capability to Evaluate Compliance with Privacy and Security Requirements

In June 2011, OCR initiated efforts to conduct pilot audits of 150 covered entities by the end of December 2012. The office contracted for a private firm to identify the population of covered entities from which to select audit candidates. Additionally, the office contracted with a private audit firm to develop the initial audit procedures for covered entities. These procedures—which OCR documentation asserts are to be in accordance with generally accepted government auditing standards[36]—are composed of the requirements from the Privacy, Security and Breach Notification Rules, which include protections afforded to prescription drug use information and uses of it for purposes other than directly providing clinical care. In January 2012, OCR officials stated that the target for audits to complete was revised to 115.

According to OCR documentation, during the pilot each audit is conducted based on the following steps:

1) An audit is initiated with the selected covered entity being informed by OCR of its selection and asked to provide documentation of its privacy, security, and breach notification compliance efforts to the contracted auditors.
2) Contracted auditors use the audit procedures developed to assess the compliance activities of the covered entity. According to officials and documentation provided, these procedures correspond to the requirements of the Privacy, Security, and Breach Notification Rules. In this pilot phase, every audit will include a documentation review and site visit.
3) Contracted auditors will provide the audited covered entity the draft findings within 30 days after conclusion of the field work.
4) Audited entities will have 10 days to provide the audit contractor with comments and outline corrective actions planned or taken.
5) Contracted auditors will develop a final audit report to submit to OCR within 30 days of receipt of the comments. The final report will describe how the audit was conducted, what the findings were, and what actions the covered entity is taking in response to those findings as well as describe any best practices of the entity.

According to OCR officials, an initial set of 20 pilot audits was completed by March 2012. Officials stated that these initial audits resulted in the identification of both privacy and security issues at covered entities, such as potential impermissible uses and disclosures and not appropriately conducting reviews of audit logs and other reports monitoring activity on information systems. OCR officials stated that the remaining 95 pilot audits, 25 of which were initiated in April 2012, will be completed by the end of December 2012.

However, OCR has yet to establish plans for (1) continuing the audit program once the audit pilot finishes in December 2012 and (2) auditing business associates for privacy and security compliance. According to OCR officials, the dedicated Recovery Act funding for the office's audit effort will expire at the end of December 2012 and officials stated that they have not yet finalized a decision on the future of the program, including the manner in which an audit process will need to be designed to address compliance by business associates.[37] OCR officials stated that the office plans to award a contract in 2012 for a review of the pilot program, including a sample of audits completed during the pilot. OCR officials anticipate that this review will help determine how the office can fully implement an audit function.

Implementing a sustained audit program could allow OCR to help covered entities and business associates identify and mitigate risks and vulnerabilities that may not be identified through OCR's current reactive processes. Furthermore, inclusion of business associates in such a program is important because, according to OCR data, more than 20 percent of data breaches affecting over 500 individuals that were reported to OCR involved business associates. Without a plan for deploying a sustained audit capability on an ongoing basis, OCR will lack the ability to ensure that covered entities and business associates are complying with HIPAA regulations, including properly de-identifying PHI when data on prescription drug use are used for purposes other than directly providing clinical care.

CONCLUSION

Through its issuance of regulations, outreach, and enforcement activities, HHS has established a framework for protecting the privacy and security of Medicare beneficiaries' prescription drug use information when used for purposes other than directly providing clinical care. It has also promoted public awareness on the uses and disclosures of PHI through its education and outreach activities. Further, OCR has established and implemented a process to enforce provisions of the HIPAA Privacy and Security Rules through investigations. However, it has not issued required implementation guidance to assist entities in de-identifying PHI. By not issuing the guidance, increased risk exists that covered entities are not properly implementing the standards set by the HIPAA Privacy Rule and that PHI is not properly stripped of all identifiers that would identify an individual. In addition, OCR has not fully established a capability to proactively monitor covered entities' compliance through the use of periodic audits as required by the HITECH Act. Specifically, OCR has yet to establish plans for a sustained audit capability upon completion of its pilot program at the end calendar year 2012 and has yet to determine how to include auditing business associates. Without a plan for deploying a sustained audit capability on an ongoing basis, OCR will have limited assurance that covered entities and business associates are complying with HIPAA regulations, including whether Medicare beneficiaries' prescription drug use information, when used for purposes other than directly providing clinical care, is being appropriately safeguarded from compromise.

Recommendations for Executive Action

To improve the department's guidance and oversight efforts for ensuring the privacy and security of protected health information, including Medicare beneficiaries' prescription drug use information, we recommend that the Secretary of HHS direct the Director of the Office for Civil Rights to take the following two actions:

- Issue guidance on properly implementing the HIPAA Privacy Rule requirements for the de-identification of protected health information.
- Establish plans for conducting periodic audits to ensure covered entities and business associates are complying with the HIPAA Privacy and Security Rules and breach notification standards.

Agency Comments and Our Evaluation

In written comments on a draft of the report, the HHS Assistant Secretary for Legislation agreed with our two recommendations, but provided qualifying comments for both.

Regarding our recommendation that OCR issue guidance on properly implementing the HIPAA Privacy Rule requirements for the de-identification of protected health information, the Assistant Secretary stated that while the department agrees that issuing the guidance will be helpful to covered entities, the department does not agree that without the guidance, covered entities will have limited assurance that they are complying with the HIPAA Privacy Rule de-identification standards. The Assistant Secretary noted that covered entities have been operating under these existing de-identification standards for almost 10 years and that OCR has not found that the standards have been the subject of significant or frequent compliance issues by covered entities. The Assistant Secretary noted that OCR's purpose in issuing the de-identification guidance was to provide covered entities with the current options and approaches available for de-identifying health information.

We agree that the existing agency information on the de-identification standards provide a level of assurance that covered entities have the parameters and requirements needed to properly remove identifiers from PHI and have clarified this in our report. However, the HITECH Act requires HHS to issue de-identification implementation guidance that addresses how covered entities should implement the de-identification standards. OCR officials stated that the planned guidance will explain and answer questions about de-identification methods as well as clarify guidelines for conducting the expert determination method of de-identification to reduce entities' reliance on the Safe Harbor method. Such information could assist covered entities in determining how to properly implement the de-identification methods. Until such implementation guidance is issued, increased risk exists that covered entities are not properly adhering to the standards set by the HIPAA Privacy Rule and that PHI is not properly stripped of all identifiers that would identify an individual.

Regarding our recommendation that OCR establish plans for conducting periodic audits to ensure covered entities and business associates are complying with the HIPAA Privacy and Security Rules and breach notification standards, the Assistant Secretary stated the department did not agree with our report's conclusion that without such a plan, OCR will lack the ability to ensure that covered entities and business associates are complying with the HIPAA rules. Specifically, he stated that our conclusion did not adequately take into account the considerable impact of the thousands of complaint investigations, compliance reviews, and other enforcement activities OCR conducts annually to ensure covered entities are complying with the rules. He noted that although the audit function is a critical compliance tool for identifying vulnerabilities, the importance of the audit function should not be understood to diminish the effectiveness of OCR's other enforcement activities for bringing about and enforcing compliance with the HIPAA rules.

As our report highlighted, OCR has developed and implemented an enforcement process that is focused on responding to actions that potentially violate the Privacy and Security Rules. OCR conducts this reactive process through processing complaints and conducting thousands of investigations each year. An audit program is an important addition to OCR's compliance program as it is a tool to identify vulnerabilities before they cause breaches and other incidents. Without the addition of a proactive process, such as an audit capability, OCR will have limited assurance that covered entities are complying with HIPAA regulations.

HHS also provided technical comments on the report draft, which we addressed in the final report as appropriate.

Gregory C. Wilshusen
Director
Information Security Issues

APPENDIX I: OBJECTIVE, SCOPE, AND METHODOLOGY

Our objective was to determine the extent to which the Department of Health and Human Services (HHS) has established a framework to ensure the privacy and security of Medicare beneficiaries' protected health information (PHI) when data on prescription drug use are used for purposes other than their direct clinical care.

To address our objective, we identified HHS's and its Office for Civil Rights' (OCR) responsibilities for protecting the privacy and security of PHI by reviewing and analyzing the Health Insurance Portability and Accountability Act (HIPAA), including the HIPAA Privacy and Security Rules; the Health Information Technology for Economic and Clinical Health (HITECH) Act; and applicable privacy best practices, such as the Fair Information Practices.

To obtain information on OCR efforts in implementing HIPAA's and the HITECH Act's requirements, we reviewed and analyzed documentation related to the office's public outreach and guidance efforts, enforcement practices, and regulations for covered entity and business associate compliance provided by the office and through the department's website and compared those documents to the office's statutory requirements. To obtain information on the office's enforcement through complaint and breach notice investigations, we interviewed officials, reviewed agency-provided and public information, and analyzed agency documentation. We conducted interviews with OCR officials to discuss the department's approaches and future plans for addressing the protection and enforcement requirements of the HIPAA Privacy and Security Rules that applied to covered entities and business associates. We also analyzed plans and documentation provided by OCR officials that described enforcement and compliance activities for developing an audit mechanism and compared them with requirements for the audit program established in the HITECH Act.

To describe the uses of prescription drug use data for purposes other than directly providing clinical care, we interviewed representatives from several covered entities, business associates, and medical associations, and reviewed the HIPAA Privacy Rule and academic publications.

We conducted this performance audit at the Department of Health and Human Services in Washington, D.C., from August 2011 through June 2012, in accordance with generally accepted government auditing standards. Those standards require that we plan and perform the audit to obtain sufficient, appropriate evidence to provide a reasonable basis for our findings and conclusions based on our audit objectives. We believe that the evidence obtained provides a reasonable basis for our findings and conclusions based on our audit objectives.

APPENDIX II: KEY PERMISSIBLE USES OF PROTECTED HEALTH INFORMATION

Permissible use	Description	Example
Treatment	The provision, coordination, or management of health care and related services among health care providers or by a health care provider with a third party, consultation between health care providers regarding a patient, or the referral of a patient from one health care provider to another.	A hospital may use protected health information about an individual to provide health care to the individual and may consult with other health care providers about the individual's treatment. A hospital may send a patient's health care instructions to a nursing home to which the patient is transferred.

(Continued)

Permissible use	Description	Example
Payment	The various activities of health care providers to obtain payment or be reimbursed for their services and of a health plan to obtain premiums, to fulfill their coverage responsibilities and provide benefits under the plan, and to obtain or provide reimbursement for the provision of health care.	A hospital emergency department may give a patient's payment information to an ambulance service provider that transported the patient to the hospital in order for the ambulance provider to bill for its service
Healthcare Operations	Certain administrative, financial, legal, and quality improvement activities of a covered entity, as defined in the Privacy Rule, that are necessary to run its business and to support the core functions of treatment and payment.	Conducting quality assessment and improvement activities, and case management and care coordination. Business management and general administrative activities, including those related to implementing and complying with the Privacy Rule.
Marketing	With certain exceptions, to make a communication about a product or service that encourages recipients of the communication to purchase or use the product or service. Marketing includes an arrangement between a covered entity and any other entity, whereby the covered entity discloses PHI to the other entity in exchange for direct or indirect remuneration, for the other entity or its affiliate to make a communication about a product or service that encourages recipients of the communication to purchase or use the product or service. With limited exceptions, such as for face to face communications, the Privacy Rule requires an individual's written authorization before a use or disclosure of his or her PHI can be made for marketing.	Needing an individual's authorization: A health plan sells a list of its members to a company that sells blood glucose monitors, which intends to send the plan's members brochures on the benefits of purchasing and using the monitors. Not needing an individual's authorization: An insurance agent sells a health insurance policy in person to a customer and proceeds to also market a casualty and life insurance policy as well
Disclosure for Public Health Activities	Covered entities may disclose protected health information, without authorization, to public health authorities who are legally authorized to receive such reports for the purpose of preventing or controlling disease, injury, or disability.	The social services department of a local government might have legal authority to receive reports of child abuse or neglect, in which case the Privacy Rule would permit a covered entity to report such cases to that authority without obtaining individual authorization.

Permissible use	Description	Example
Research	A systematic investigation, including research development, testing, and evaluation, designed to develop or contribute to generalizable knowledge. To use or disclose protected health information without authorization by the research participant, a covered entity must obtain either: (1) institutional review board or privacy board waiver of authorization; (2) representations for a preparatory to research activity; (3) representations that the research is on the protected health information of decedents; or (4) a data use agreementa with recipient where only a limited data setsb is shared.	Approval of a waiver of authorization by an Institutional Review Board or Privacy Board for research, such as for certain records research, when the Board has determined that the use or disclosure of protected health information involves no more than a minimal risk to the privacy of individuals, and the research could not practicably be conducted without the waiver and without access to the protected health informat

Source: HHS Office for Civil Rights.

[a] A covered entity may always use or disclose for research purposes health information which has been de-identified.

[b] A limited data set excludes specified direct identifiers of the individual or of relatives, employers, or household members of the individual.

End Notes

[1] Pub. L. No. 110-275, § 132(c), 122 Stat. 2494, 2527-2531 (July 15, 2008).

[2] MIPPA also required us to report on aspects of the Electronic Prescribing Program, which we fulfilled in GAO, *Electronic Prescribing: CMS Should Address Inconsistencies in Its Two Incentive Programs That Encourage the Use of Health Information Technology*, GAO-11-159 (Washington, D.C.: Feb. 17, 2011).

[3] A formulary is a list of generic and brand name prescription drugs, grouped by therapeutic class.

[4] Individually identifiable health information is information, including demographic information collected from an individual, that (1) is created or received by a health care provider, health plan, employer, or health care clearinghouse; (2) relates to the past, present, or future physical or mental health or condition of the individual or the provision of or payment for health care to the individual; and (3) can be used to identify the individual or with respect to which there is a reasonable basis to believe the information can be used to identify the individual. 45 C.F.R. § 160.103.

[5] Protected health information is individually identifiable health information that is transmitted or maintained in any form or medium, and in this report it is used interchangeably with individually identifiable health information.

[6] Covered entities are defined under regulations implementing HIPAA as health plans that provide or pay for the medical care of individuals, health care providers that electronically transmit health information in connection with transactions covered by the regulations, and

health care clearinghouses that receive health information from other entities and process or facilitate the processing of that information into standard or nonstandard format for those entities (45 C.F.R. § 160.103).

[7] An electronic health record is a collection of information about the health of an individual or the care provided, including patient demographics, progress notes, problems, medications, vital signs, past medical history, immunizations, laboratory data, and radiology reports.

[8] Medicare's Part D provides outpatient prescription drug benefits for Medicare beneficiaries.

[9] Pub. L. No. 104-191, Title II, Subtitle F, 110 Stat. 1936, 2021 (codified at 42 U.S.C. §§ 1320d–1320d-8). The HIPAA Privacy and Security Rules were promulgated at 45 C.F.R. Parts 160 and 164.

[10] The HITECH Act was enacted as Title XIII of Division A and Title IV of Division B of the American Recovery and Reinvestment Act. Pub. L. No. 111-5, Div. A, Tit. XIII, 123 Stat. 115, 226-279 and Div. B, Tit. IV, 123 Stat. 115, 467-496 (Feb. 17, 2009).

[11] HHS is the federal government's principal agency responsible for protecting the health of Americans, including Medicare beneficiaries.

[12] The Administrative Simplification Provisions of HIPAA provided for the establishment of national standards for the electronic transmission of certain health information, such as standards for certain health care transactions conducted electronically and code sets and unique health care identifiers for health care providers and employers.

[13] HIPAA establishes civil money penalties and criminal penalties for violations. 42 U.S.C. §§ 1320d-5-1320d-6. HHS enforces the civil money penalties, while the Department of Justice enforces the criminal penalties. If a complaint is received about a covered entity that describes an action that could be a violation of the criminal provisions of HIPAA, it may be referred to the Department of Justice for investigation.

[14] The Secretary of HHS issued the HIPAA Privacy Rule in December 2000, and it was amended in August 2002. The initial compliance date for the HIPAA Privacy Rule was April 2003 for most covered entities.

[15] There are exceptions to the "minimum necessary" requirement of the Privacy Rule for certain disclosures for treatment and uses and disclosures required by law.

[16] The 18 unique types of identifiers are names; all geographic subdivisions smaller than a state (e.g., street address, ZIP code); Social Security numbers; account numbers; device identifiers and serial numbers; biometric identifiers, such as fingerprints and voice prints; telephone numbers; fax numbers; medical record numbers; certificate/license numbers; web uniform resource locators (URLs); full-face photographic images and any comparable images; all dates that are related to an individual (e.g., date of birth, admission); e-mail addresses; health plan beneficiary numbers; vehicle identifiers and serial numbers, including license plate numbers; Internet protocol (IP) address numbers; and any other unique identifying numbers, characteristics, or codes.

[17] 45 C.F.R. §§ 164.302-164.318. The initial compliance date for the HIPAA Security Rule was April 2005 for most covered entities.

[18] An interim final rule is a final rule that has the full force and effect of law; thus, affected parties have an obligation to comply with its requirements. An interim final rule allows stakeholders to submit comments during the public comment period on the areas requested in the interim final rule that the agency will consider before deciding whether to issue a revised final rule or confirm the interim final rule as final.

[19] 74 Fed. Reg. 42740 (Aug. 24, 2009).

[20] 74 Fed. Reg. 56123 (Oct. 30, 2009).

[21] A breach is generally an impermissible use or disclosure under the Privacy Rule that compromises the security or privacy of the PHI such that the use or disclosure poses a significant risk of financial, reputational, or other harm to the affected individual.

[22] 75 Fed. Reg. 40868 (July 14, 2010).

[23] The guidance issued by OCR applies generally to all PHI and the various HIPAA requirements for safeguarding PHI, restricting its use and disclosure, providing individuals their rights with respect to their PHI, and other administrative requirements. As such, the guidance would apply to Medicare beneficiaries' prescription drug use information used for purposes other than direct clinical care.

[24] OCR guidance and educational outreach materials can be found at this site: http://www.hhs.gov/ocr/privacy/.

[25] The Office of the National Coordinator for Health Information Technology is a component of the Office of the Secretary of HHS. Its primary focus is on the coordination of nationwide efforts to implement and use health information technology and the electronic exchange of health information.

[26] The Privacy and Security Framework is focused on establishing a policy framework for electronic health information exchange that can help guide the nation's adoption of health information technologies and help improve the availability of health information and health care quality.

[27] As previously discussed, de-identification involves the removal of PHI (e.g., name, date of birth, and Social Security number) that can be used to identify an individual.

[28] The Privacy and Security Rules established the ability for individuals to file complaints with the department if they believed that a covered entity was not complying with a provision of the rules.

[29] Pub. L. No. 111-5, § 13411, 123 Stat. 115, 276.

[30] Complaints present an eligible case for enforcement by OCR if they meet certain criteria: (1) the alleged action must have taken place after April 13, 2003, for a Privacy Rule complaint, and after April 19, 2005, for a Security Rule complaint; (2) the complaint must be filed against an entity that is required by law to comply with the Privacy and Security Rules; (3) a complaint must allege an activity that, if proven true, would violate the Privacy or Security Rule; and (4) complaints must be filed within 180 days of when the person knew or should have known about the alleged violation (OCR may waive this time limit if it determines that there was "good cause" for not submitting the complaint within 180 days).

[31] Data breach notification investigations, according to OCR officials, are initiated for every breach affecting 500 or more individuals; for breaches affecting under 500 individuals, notifications are provided to the regional investigation offices which determine if the breach warrants an investigation.

[32] OCR has received Privacy Rule complaints since April 14, 2003, and Security Rule complaints since October 2009.

[33] The majority of complaints received by OCR were related to potential violations of the Privacy Rule.

[34] U.S. Department of Health and Human Services Office for Civil Rights, "Annual Report to Congress on HIPAA Privacy Rule and Security Rule Compliance For Calendar Years 2009 and 2010," Washington, D.C.: Aug. 11, 2011.

[35] The four categories of culpability for purposes of imposing civil money penalties are (1) did not know, (2) reasonable cause, (3) willful neglect—corrected, and (4) willful neglect— not corrected.

[36] Audits that are conducted in accordance with generally accepted government auditing standards can provide an independent, objective, nonpartisan assessment of individual entities' compliance with the relevant federal laws and regulations.

[37] According to OCR officials, business associate compliance was not an element of the pilot program because changes to the regulations to implement the HITECH Act amendments extending liability for compliance to business associates would not be in effect during the period of the audit pilot program.

INDEX

D

E

P

Q

R

S